The Maya Method

Easy & Simple Chair Yoga
Exercises For Weight Loss,
Increased Energy & Happiness

Florence Gauthier
David O'Connor

© **Copyright 2024 - All rights reserved.**

The content contained within this book may not be reproduced, duplicated, or transmitted without direct written permission from the author or the publisher.

Under no circumstances will any blame or legal responsibility be held against the publisher, or author, for any damages, reparation, or monetary loss due to the information contained within this book, either directly or indirectly.

Legal Notice:

This book is copyright protected. It is only for personal use. You cannot amend, distribute, sell, use, quote, or paraphrase any part, or the content within this book, without the consent of the author or publisher.

Disclaimer Notice:

Please note the information contained within this document is for educational and entertainment purposes only. All effort has been executed to present accurate, up-to-date, reliable, and complete information. No warranties of any kind are declared or implied. Readers acknowledge that the author is not engaged in the rendering of legal, financial, medical, or professional advice. The content within this book has been derived from various sources. Please consult a licensed professional before attempting any techniques outlined in this book.

By reading this document, the reader agrees that under no circumstances is the author responsible for any losses, direct or indirect, that are incurred as a result of the use of the information contained within this document, including, but not limited to, errors, omissions, or inaccuracies.

TABLE OF CONTENTS

Foreword 9
Introduction 13
   How to Use This Book 16
Chapter 1: Mostly Sane, Maybe Not! 19
Chapter 2: A Freefall in My Own Eyes 27
Chapter 3: Jane! 33
Chapter 4: On a Rampage Anytime, Anywhere 39
Chapter 5: Reigning in, Finally! 50
   My Practice 53
Chapter 6: Stumbling Upon Surprises 59
   On Why I Have Been Reluctant to Do Yoga 62
   On Activity (Surprise, Surprise!) 63
   On Designing My Days 65
   I Am Showing Progress 67

Chapter 7: Are We Afraid of Change? 70
   The Elephant and the Rider. 72
   My Relationship With Food. 73
   Notes on My Lifestyle 78
   The Act of Being Seated 81
   I Am Finally Making Headway. 82

Chapter 8: Bold and Beautiful Experiments 83
   When Negative Becomes Positive. 85
   Over the Next Few Weeks 89

Chapter 9: Picking up Threads 93
   June: New work–life balance 93
   My Little Breakthroughs 97

Chapter 10: Losing It With Love .102
   On Designing My Days 105
   On How Exercise Affects the Brain 106
   Not Forgetting to Love Oneself .107
   What I Learned About Body Fat. 111
   On Why High-Intensity Interval Training (HIIT)
   Works Well and the Science Behind It 112
   My Introduction to HIIT. 113

Chapter 11: Looking for the Perfect Recipe. 114
   The Essential Ingredients of a Fitness Plan 117
   The Chicken or Egg Story: Weight or Metabolism?. . . . 119
   On the Mistakes I Have Been Making
   When Exercising. 121

Chapter 12: Gain Without Pain—I'm Loving It! 123
   My Initiation to the Squeaky New World
   of Resistance Bands 126
   Why Having Strength Becomes More Important
   as We Grow Older 130
   I Refuse to Exclude Pleasure From Exercise 131

Chapter 13: The Scroll 133
   Why Bother With Warm-Ups 134
   What to Be Cautious of During Chair Yoga 134
Maya's Video Library 136
   Complimentary Access 136
Postures How-To 137
   The Mountain Pose and Its Variations (Tadasana) 137
      Mountain Posture on the Chair #1 137
      Mountain Pose With Side Stretch
      (Tiryaka Tadasana) #2 140
      Back Bound Mountain Pose
      (Baddha Hasta Tadasana) #3 142
   The Raised Hand Pose and Its Variations
   (Urdhava Hastasana) 144
      Raised Hands Pose #4 144
      Crescent Moon on the Chair
      (Parsva Urdhva Hastasana) #5 146
   The Tree Pose (Vrikshasana) 148
      The Standing Tree Pose #6 148
   The Cat-Cow Pose (Marjaryasana-Bitilasana) 150
      The Cat-Cow Stretch on the Floor #7 150
      Chair Cat-Cow (Marjaryasana-Bitilasana) #8 152

- The Forward Fold Pose and Its Variations (Uttanasana) 154
  - Half Forward-Fold (Ardha Uttanasana) #9 154
  - Forward Fold Pose on the Chair (Uttanasana) #10 156
  - Standing Forward Fold (Uttanasana) #11 158
  - The Crescent Lunge (Anjaneyasana) #12 160
  - Happy Baby Pose (Upavistha Ardha Ananda Balasana) #13 162
  - Head to Knee Pose (Parivrtta Janu Sirsasana) #14 164
  - Marichi Pose (Marichyasana) #15 166
  - Sun Salutation (Suryanamaskar) #16 168
  - Cobra Pose (Bhujangasana) #17 170
  - Dolphin Pose (Ardha Pincha Mayurasana) #18 172
  - Hand-to-Toes (Hasta Padangusthasana) #19 174
  - Hand-to-Toes Variation With Strap #20 176
  - Easy Pose (Sukhasana) #21 178
  - Lion Pose (Simhasana) #22 180
  - Chin Lock Pose (Jalandhara Bandha) #23 182
- The Downward Dog Pose and Its Variations 184
  - Downward Dog on the Chair (Adho Mukha Svanasana) #24 184
  - Wide-Legged Downward Dog Pose (Prasarita Adho Mukha Svanasana) #25 186
  - The Downward Dog on the Floor (Adho Mukha Svanasana) #26 188
  - Three-Legged Downward Dog (Tri Pada Adho Mukha Svanasana) #27 190

The Warrior Pose and Its Variations................193
   The Warrior 1 Pose (Virabhadrasana 1) #28.......193
   The Warrior 2 Pose (Virabhadrasana 2) #29......196
The Plank Poses.....................................198
   Plank Pose on Chair (Phalakasana) #30..........198
   Upward Plank Pose
   (Upavistha Purvottanasana) #31................200
Four-Limbed Staff Pose
(Chaturanga Dandasana)...................... 202
   Variation 1 #32................................ 202
   Variation 2 #33................................ 204
   Triangle Pose (Trikonasana) #34................ 206
   Revolved Triangle Pose
   (Parivrtta Trikonasana) #35..................... 208
High Lunge Pose and Its Variations.................210
   High Lunge Pose With a Chair
   (Ashta Chandrasana) #36......................210
   High Lunge Variation (Ashta Chandrasana) #37...212
   High Lunge Non-Chair
   (Ashta Chandrasana) #38......................214
   Upward-Facing Dog Pose
   (Urdhva Mukha Svanasana) #39 216
   Goddess Pose Side Stretch
   (Utkata Konasana) #40........................218
   Bharadvaja's Twist (Bharadvajasana) #41......... 220
   Half-Fish Pose (Ardha Matsyendrasana) #42......222
   Vishnu's Couch Pose (Ananthasana) #43 224
   Half Frog Pose (Ardha Bhekasana) #44..........226

- Half Frog Variation With a Strap #45 228
- Pyramid Pose (Parsvottanasana) #46 229
- Dancer's Pose (Natarajasana) #47 232
- The Garland Pose (Malasana) and Its Variations 234
  - Seated Garland Pose (Upavistha Malasana) #48 .. 235
  - Garland Pose Hands-On Chair Support (Malasana Hasta) #49 237
  - Garland Pose With Towel, Blocks, or a Partner #50 239
  - Garland Pose (Malasana) #51 241
  - Garland Half Broken Wing Pose (Malasana Ardha Avabhinna Pakshasana) #52 243
  - Revolved Chair Pose (Parivrtta Utkatasana) #53 ... 245
  - Revolved Chair Pose Variation (Parivrtta Utkatasana Variation) #54 248
  - Half Moon Pose on Chair (Ardha Chandrasana) #55 250
  - Sugarcane Bow Pose on Chair (Ardha Chandra Chapasana) #56 253
  - Bound Angle and Seated Upward Straddle Pose (Baddha Konasana and Urdhva Upavistha Konasana) #57 255
- Conclusion 258

FOREWORD

Florence and I wanted to go further than simply provide yet another Chair yoga book! We have our yoga class members to thank for the inspired idea of combining a 'full' chair yoga guide (50+ illustrated poses) with a fictional story. We asked what would have benefited them when starting yoga at home, assuming no knowledge of body alignment, breathing techniques or yoga poses. Their answer: someone to offer encouragement, who appreciated the difficulties they faced. Our hope is that you will find Maya's story, of a busy women juggling career and family commitments whilst trying to find 'me' time to devote to her wellness, relatable. Maya will be your co-traveller, talking to you and mirroring your fears and triumphs. She will inspire, transform, engage, and encourage you, empathize with your frustrations and celebrate your breakthroughs as you embark upon your chair yoga journey.

    We also want to ensure you have access to a 'human' narrated audiobook (the need to specify 'human' seems odd but with so many books offering low quality AI voices it's worth pointing out) as well as DVD quality instructional videos. So no matter how you find it easiest to learn this book has you covered (at no additional cost!)

The Maya Method is for anyone starting out, irrespective of age, as most poses are beginner level but for those more advanced, Maya has included modifications and some to challenge even experienced practitioners.

Whether you choose to jump straight to the detailed pose instructions or read Maya's story first, we hope you'll enjoy the physical and mental benefits chair yoga can offer.

Florence and David

COMPLIMENTARY MATERIALS TO HELP YOU ACHIEVE YOUR GOALS

To ensure you gain the maximum benefit from The Maya Method we have included free access to:

- The **audiobook**. Simply scan a QR code to listen to a chapter or a specific pose 'How-To' instructions. The beautifully narrated audio is a great companion, you don't have to open the book and our students report that it helps them focus and maintain motivation.
- **Maya's video library.** You have lifetime access to Maya's video library containing 50+ specifically recorded videos to accompany this book. If you are unsure how to perform an asana, video can play an important role in helping you achieve the correct movement and body alignment. Each video is narrated, explaining clearly the movement sequence required to perfect the pose! **Simply follow the instructions on page 136.**

or for a sneak preview

SCAN QR CODE

- We've put together five of **Maya's favorite yoga sequences** (flows) for you to try!
    - Early morning/waking flow
    - Seated office flow
    - Energy and strength flow
    - Anytime energizer flow
    - Before bed relaxation flow

- **Resistance Band and HIIT Workout Book.** For those wishing to accelerate the achievement of their yoga goals download your complimentary copy (pdf or ebook formats).

SCAN FOR A FREE BONUS

INTRODUCTION

SCAN FOR AUDIO CHAPTER

Maya must clearly define her relationship with her body if she wants to make it function on her terms.

Losing excess fat and bringing our fitness and energy to stellar levels is a fabulous idea. Imagine feeling and looking good, being admired for the aura we create wherever we go, doing a dream trek, fitting into a terrific suit, and being picked for a challenging project at work simply because we ooze confidence in whatever we do. Life would be so much more satisfying.

Having said that, we should not forget that we've been raised in societies influenced by industries that promote certain body images and push us to emulate them. To make matters worse, this achievement is touted to be synonymous with success and happiness!

Our boxed notions of an ideal weight and body measurement result in us asking for the impossible; we willingly fall again and again for the mirage that eludes us. So, right here, right now, promise yourself that you want to be your best self, not somebody else's definition of your best self, and dive into Maya's captivating story.

This whirlwind tale is of an ambitious corporate lawyer, mother, and empathetic confidante who is brilliant, ambitious, and hugely successful in her career yet vulnerable to deeply hidden fears of self-worth. Maya finds the voices of aging and body image issues growing louder within her by the day and begins to perceive signs of them in her colleagues, friends, and family. Irrespective of age, sex, or social standing, they are all fighting the same battle as she is, whether they admit to it or not.

Following a casual, rather well-intentioned comment from an old acquaintance, Maya's hazy realizations and underlying turmoil explode into a rage and morph into an intense curiosity that gets her to finally face her fears. This, followed by the desire to crack the code, if there was one, leads to Maya collecting wisdom that leaves her stunned. The answers come from the most unexpected sources and in the most unimaginable forms. They are hard-hitting, not because they are complex and elusive but because they are so simple and elegant. In the noise, Maya finds hidden peace; in the clutter, she discovers a gem.

The ordinary process of finding the extraordinary allows her to experience childlike joy, a spring in her steps, and compassion for herself and society once again. She also gets to fit into that designer dress and is still the go-to legal eagle at the chambers!

This book will be your co-traveler, talking to you and mirroring your fears and triumphs. It will inspire, transform, engage, and encourage you. It will empathize with your frustrations and celebrate your breakthroughs. It will also provide insights into why incorporating a fitness schedule into your busy life is challenging and how you can get around this by coming up with creative solutions. We need to develop clever hacks to take care of the foggy, ever-transforming fitness predicaments of jet-setters.

Get to know Maya, a zealous corporate attorney in her late 30s living in New York City, through her intense private thoughts and crazy busy life. Maya is surrounded by people who all want to live life to the fullest when it comes to their professional aspirations, personal development, and family commitments, and they all have challenges with balancing work and life.

It helps that Maya is charmingly eclectic and has a curious mind that understands and processes information from everything she senses. She will help us dissect the psychological, emotional, social, and professional barriers we all face and will most certainly inspire each one of us to build an actionable fitness regimen. She will also help us explore and examine the faulty ideas put into our minds by the fitness industry and prompt us to push back and ask the right questions.

HOW TO USE THIS BOOK

We invite you to reflect on the anecdotes and ideas woven into the narrative of this book, which represents you and me, individuals influenced by cultures of the contemporary world. It will most certainly help you relate to the situations and own them. We'd love you to contemplate Maya's observations; discernments on health, food, body image, the many urban myths we consume, and our attitudes about designing our lives; and the actions she initiates that help her take charge of her life. You can get to the crux of self-care by cutting the clutter from random sources in the form of self-help tips. We are sure you will find your "*Aha!*" moments alongside Maya.

This book aims to make you fall in love with yoga, but it also wants to take you further: With your new yoga mindset, you will begin to appreciate the other good things in life.

We have curated a dynamic set of in-depth chair and floor yoga techniques along with clever sequencing to seamlessly fit into a busy work schedule.

For once, the instructions are written from the learner's perspective, empathizing with how a novice would look at them: skeptical and full of questions in the mind and heart.

We will also delve into the realm of food. With growing confusion around the right ways of eating, polarized views on food, and concerns about new psychological conditions and eating disorders (The latest buzz being orthorexia), the dialogue is inevitable.

In addition to cultivating the right mindset to help manage our environment for a win-win situation, this book will help deliver excuse-proof solutions that empathize with the harsh demands of our work and life. Promise yourself that you will not use this book to just look at someone else's life but to live and experience your version of the bumps and triumphs of the protagonist. After all, this is about you!

Follow Maya's point of view to get a common person's perspective of what it means to incorporate seemingly alien and sometimes intimidating ideas of changing one's lifestyle. Through her shaky start and eventual discovery of peace, you will find the thrill of overcoming skepticism.

The How-To instructions and the illustrations in "The Scroll" will be your guide to gaining control of your workout patterns and poses. It will speak to you about the nuances and pitfalls. These practical lessons will be the teacher you have been keen on having around. It will take you through the meaning of yoga and the reasons for the popularity of chair workouts among busy people. Moreover, the progression of exercises will help you sustain the practice for decades to come.

We invite you to savor each pose and workout at an unhurried pace. Each of them takes time to internalize, and the practice goes from superficial to deep absorption every time you reach out to it. What's more, you can easily switch between reading and listening by scanning the QR codes to access a human-narrated **audiobook version** of the text—it'll be like having your very own yoga instructor!

CHAPTER 1

MOSTLY SANE, MAYBE NOT!

SCAN FOR AUDIO CHAPTER

1:45 p.m. on a typical day at work

Meryl, my intern, gasped at the aggression in my tone. I had a briefing at 2 p.m. but did not yet have the documents on my table. I had wolfed down my sandwich in two bites and was good to go, but Meryl didn't seem to care.

"She just doesn't know what needs to be done!" I muttered to myself, seething.

I wanted to yank the file out of Meryl's hands and walk out the door, forcing her to scamper after me, but I knew better.

7:00 p.m. back at home

I sat on the couch, physically and emotionally exhausted, and I could feel the energy draining from my body. The meeting had gone well, but I had a bad feeling. I was unsure what this strong emotion was and dared not attempt to describe it in words. A sense of defeat was overcoming me, but I refused to acknowledge it.

My daughter, Hazel, burst through the door, squealing with delight that I was home, and wanted me to have a piece of the cake she'd gotten from kindergarten today. I reluctantly took a nibble and saw her face change. She was annoyed. I got on the defensive and tried to explain "Thank you, baby, for saving me a piece, but you know cake is not healthy for Mamma."

That did nothing to erase her annoyance. I sighed and accepted that I had disappointed her.

"How was your day, darling?" I asked in all earnest, hoping to change the topic.

"Fine."

Then, Hazel's eyes softened at the sight of her toys, while mine grew heavier. I listened to her play with her toys for a bit before falling asleep, taking a well-earned early evening snooze.

8:00 p.m. I spring off the couch

My eyes flew open—there was so much to do! I was famished but needed to fix up Hazel's dinner and get her to bed on time. She could get cranky when tired, and I was in no mood for tantrums. I had promised to tell her a bedtime story today but couldn't think of one. Nolan would be on his way back from the airport, and both of us needed to get back to work the next day—the week had just begun! Also, if only I could get a little time to browse through The Gazette before I hit the bed, it could help me have an edge at the hearing tomorrow—if only I could go for a stroll in the garden too. I have been meaning to do that for quite a long time now.

9:00 a.m. the next morning

I was at the office, feeling cheery because I had the case under control. It appeared like it would be my day at the hearing. I had caught up on my sleep well past midnight. Hazel had finally dozed off, not before declaring Daddy to be a better storyteller. Nolan and I had a late dinner and finally made time for a stroll in the garden—after eons! Six hours of sleep was not exactly restful for me, but I needed a couple of hours in the morning to finalize the contract. I had hit the snooze button one too many times but gotten ready in 12 minutes flat. Well, it has become my ritual of sorts.

12:00 p.m. lunchtime

Meryl was sorting papers robotically. I was nearly repentant for having been impatient with her the day before, but I couldn't brush off the annoyance of her perpetual unhurried demeanor. She should be more agile—she's 20-something for heaven's sake! Instead, she takes her time soaking in the chatter while she sips coffee and eats lunch, proceeding with any research and never-ending deliberations with irritating nonchalance. I could not, however, point fingers at any carelessness or lack of initiative. She had the same efficiency and drive as any other intern, and she was charming and stylish. She had that "been there, done that—I have it figured out" vibe about her as if she already had the answers I was desperately seeking; my mind would race every time I saw her. I only knew that something about her triggered me. I even felt guilty about it.

7:00 p.m. winding up the day

I had a few minutes to myself. I preferred to wait till the parking lot got calmer. I sat in the empty chambers and looked out the window. From my soundproof office on the 27th floor, Manhattan and beyond looked like an ocean of lights as peaceful as the stars in the sky. Little did it reflect the noise and chaos of the people who made the city what it was—all the vehicles were heading home.

I would be hitting 37 this year and thought about how I had already put in a ton of work, established my niche in the legal field, and was content at having realized many of my dreams. Being unapologetically ambitious and stumbling through impossible work hours with the house, husband, and kid in tow has been a roller coaster ride.

Having been born in downtown Chicago to very hardworking parents, I knew I couldn't avoid discipline if I had to add meaning to my work and personal life. In actively pursuing my career, I was playing my part and aware of being an inspiration to many around me. The fundamentals were right, so to speak, but what was that vague emptiness nagging me? Was it a mid-life crisis? What's that supposed to mean in any case? Is it something that would pass on its own? I hoped it would.

The week zipped past in any case. My hands were too full to have time to brood on anything that was not specific. I needed to catch up on some sleep, and as always, I promised myself I would.

It was not that I was unaware of my changing personality. In my teens and 20s, I was athletic and a quirky mix of enchanting and coming across as a livewire. I had my share of mess-ups and did quite a bit of experimenting with my life and looks. I was always image-conscious, often getting into and out of diets and swinging between months of inactivity and bouts of mind-blowing physical exertions. My body too seemed to lend itself happily to my whims.

I was nonchalant. I had my way of impressing guys and was the ideal student for teachers. So, my parents did not have to fret about where I was heading. I would lend an ear to my friends coping with weight issues and self-worth troubles and learn along the way. Graduation had me hooked on exams, internships, and the race for prestigious placements, However, it did not stop me from experiencing all life had to offer—music, movies, gadgets, friends, sports, fashion, politics, gossip, travel, love affairs, and everything in between!

Now, my life is very different. With so much on my calendar, I became more sedentary, and my once-toned body transformed into a soft, flabby figure. My hair was thinner, and the scale brought no joy. However, the adulation and authority that came with being professionally successful and having a dreamlike family made me feel guilty about complaining.

The following week was unusual. Nolan had taken a few days off to visit his parents in Canada and was taking Hazel along. I knew Hazel would be happy and well looked after. I was glad she could be apart from me without any hassle. Nolan and I were fully functional parents and clear about raising a strong independent girl capable of communicating her feelings.

They left on Friday evening. After the scramble of shopping, packing, and the see-offs, I fell into reset mode. It dawned on me that I had the entire weekend and the following week to myself. Though it was a long-planned trip, I was too busy to comprehend the reality of it. I had mixed feelings about being left alone and having time for myself. A million plans were racing through my head. I would have the luxury of getting extra sleep, visiting a spa, going over to Elayne's to see her baby, catching up on all the back-burner tasks at the office, and skimming through the journals piling up at work.

Perhaps I caught the school-girl excitement; all I can say is that I did nothing I had planned. Throughout the week, I slept less than normal, got hooked on Netflix, and indulged in ordering in because there was no pressure to cook healthy meals for Hazel. The days trudged by with work as usual, and the evenings went by lazily despite all that planning.

I could not seem to get over the inertia. Did Netflix entertain me? Nope. It did the opposite. I felt deeply inadequate every time I saw the hourglass-figured, sophisticated leads in the series as if they had unfairly grabbed what belonged to me. I wanted to be them—it was my right, but I could only see obstacles on my path to get there. Alright, I am showing signs of burnout, but the real question is, "How can I get out of this state?"

12:00 p.m. lunch break at the office

"Hey, Tracy! What's for lunch today?" I teased. "Leaves," she said, humoring me. Tracy was called the Jillian Michaels of Griffin

Law Chambers. She was fabulously fit for a 50-year-old and a sweetheart. The only trouble was that if she was not talking business, she was talking health to the point of obsession. Her attempts to draw us into a fitness conversation had become predictable and we'd all scatter in different directions, suddenly remembering urgent work.

People would feel super conscious about eating when she was around, and she would invariably make a comment, or at least a frown, to convey her thoughts about the nutritional value of the meal. I must admit that everyone around her secretly admired- her, but her overenthusiastic and unsolicited advice put people off.

However, Tracy's kids are away at university, she is a veteran at work, and she has all the time in the world, which is in stark contrast to my chaotic days as a young mother... she could not be my role model, I decided for the hundredth time as I sat at my desk typing away frantically with multiple screens open.

"All that is fine. But what about you?" I heard a voice in my head as I leaned back to give my aching back some rest. What about me? "Well, it is not that I am ignorant or that I don't know what to do. I am just swamped with work and family and feel helpless at the moment," I argued. Over the years, I have been trying diets, gyms, yoga... everything. It's just that my schedule and my moods never allowed me to see them through, and I gave up before I even realized it.

"The firm insists that Maya Cash take up this brief." Joel Sanders-Brown, the Managing Partner of Griffin Law Chambers, where I was a Senior Associate, was talking to Dennis when I entered the corner office in the morning. "Ah, there you are! Get on this brief, Maya. You have the entire New York team at your disposal. We cannot afford to mess up on this one. Just make sure the fangs are out."

By the end of the day, strategies were drawn up, work was delegated to the 17-member team, the heat was up, and the guns were blazing. I loved days like these. They would get my blood rushing, and I would let myself get drawn into the madness. I was ruthless at getting work done, and I could sense the effect I had on people. The rush of being in charge was addictive—no wonder some people go to any length to experience it!

However, this time, a sense of detachment was tainting the exhilarating feeling. Even if it wasn't obvious, it was there nevertheless. Shaking it off, I got back to work; there was so much to do, and I looked forward to completing the assignment.

Sanders-Brown was the heart of the firm, the dream boss, and my undisputed role model. Under his deft hands, the firm had grown into one of the most admired places to work with offices in New York, Atlanta, and Massachusetts.

He was now 72 and would often say he deserved to take it easy, threatening to retire. The days he came to the New York office were all about extended lunch meetings. He bonded with the staff and caught up with the developments over limitless supplies of bagels, mozzarella sticks, and cake that were all washed down with Coke, his favorite drink. Griffin's was a second home to us, with a large part of our hearts invested here.

CHAPTER 2

A FREEFALL IN MY OWN EYES

SCAN FOR AUDIO CHAPTER

5:00 p.m. a surprising email

I was in a particularly peppy mood on Friday evening. The initial defense we'd prepared was taking shape and looking good. Nolan and Hazel were back with goodies after an exciting week.

I was scrolling aimlessly that evening when I noticed an email from my former law school about a reunion. In the 15 years since my graduation, I never got the chance to return. I was passively part of the social media class groups and actively in touch with just two of my classmates. Life was tugging me in all directions, and I realized I had weaned away both emotionally and geographically. Now, I am not sure whether it was the confidence of success—knowing people from my past would look at me with envy, sending me on an egoistic trip—or the fact that the pandemic had changed lives and perspectives with wanting to hold on to the people we knew and loved or both these feelings put together that was making me look at this reunion invite in a new light. I stared at the mail and knew I had to make this trip, no questions asked. "Chicago, here I come!" I had a good four weeks' notice.

    I was exhilarated at the thought of going back. The young student in me was resurfacing as I visualized my old friends. Would Sam be as talkative, would Sarah still flirt with any guy she saw—who is where and doing what… I so wanted to be back with my friends. I refused to believe I had been cut off from them all this while. What would I wear for the two days we would spend at the reunion? My mind kept racing, and Nolan had to put up with my law school chatter for the next few days, but he was relieved that I was taking a break.

    "I'm happy you actually decided to attend. It will energize you," he told me. He was the kind of person who wouldn't even consider missing out on meeting up with old friends. I had attended all his reunions and kept in touch more with his friends than mine.

    "You are such a sweetheart," I gushed.

    "That I am," he shrugged and grinned.

    I went shopping later that evening, keen on nailing a certain look for the occasion. I walked into the boutiques and picked up the designs I had in mind. With every trial, it began dawning on me that the clothes weren't fitting me the way I would have wished they would. The mirror presented a different picture, a far cry from my dream looks. I began losing patience. I was being overly critical, I kept reminding myself. I liked to be smartly dressed, and my office wear was all carefully tailored. After hours of trying out dresses and suits, I settled for a few pieces with the help of the consultant at the store. She was more positive than I was, and I finally got out with some good choices. The ever-lingering feeling of being out of shape, however, was accentuated in my mind even more strongly now.

November: School reunion, Chicago

Memories came rushing in as my car approached the long winding road leading away from the city toward the campus. The familiar smell of the green ash trees and the same old pattern of wind hitting my face as we picked up speed had me feeling nostalgic. I had checked into a hotel in the city and would meet everyone at six in the evening at the auditorium. Last I heard, most of the class of 2007 had confirmed their presence.

I reached the auditorium in time to see everyone trickling into the front lawns of the grand old building that was our home for five years. On the chilly November evening, with shrieks and hugs, we greeted each other, taking a few seconds each to associate the old identities with the new. We were a mixed bag: some just the same, some unrecognizable! The years had added good and not-so-good marks on each of us. We were so thrilled to be back together.

The auditorium opened, welcoming us to the grand decor. Old country music thrummed faintly while the stage mics were checked with zestful urgency. The aroma of the food together with the fragrance of the flowers created a very family-wedding-like ambience. I spotted Professor Wilson overlooking the arrangements with the student committee in full action. I was moved at the sight of him; my teacher, who not so long ago was young and brimming with electric energy but was now bearing a subdued, aging yet wisdom-filled frame. I needed some time to process this change...

After the action-filled greeting and chatter, we all finally settled into our chairs to soak in the rest of the evening. I was seated at the table with Cindy, Joh, and Ann, catching up on everything: our work, the cities we lived in, our families, and the latest sensational news. We used to bump into each other every hour for five straight years, and now, we were inaccessible to each other, which seemed unfair.

I suddenly noticed Bitul walking toward us; she had perhaps just walked in. Bitul Sen and I were well-known academic rivals. We were at each other's throats in getting the best grades, winning mock court battles, and grabbing coveted titles. I kept track of her work and knew she was hugely successful in Chicago. Part of my subconscious always saw her as my benchmark for career progression. She was as stunning as ever and single, loved the limelight, and was all over social media, carrying fashion and intellectual capabilities with finesse. I never missed any news about her, though we lived miles away from each other.

I wasn't proud of my compulsive urge to keep tabs on Bitul's successes, and I did not want to admit to being insecure.

Needless to say, I resented her or, you could say, was jealous of her. She was center stage this evening too. Unlike how I chose to settle down at a table, she chose to be out and about, chatting with everyone she met and engaging in small talk.

"Maya!" she exclaimed, coming toward me with a spontaneous lengthening in her stride. "My old-time inspiration!" She was clearly elated. I was rather flattered, knowing well that she spoke from her heart. It made me feel small for being threatened by her presence tonight.

"How have you been, sweetheart? You just disappeared into the horizon!" She exclaimed with her familiar husky, girlish voice.

"Yeah, not really," I answered, my voice sounding annoyingly impish at least to myself. "I am in New York with work and family."

"Super glad to hear that. And I am happy to see more of Maya now!" She said, looking at me head to toe. She then hugged me and began chatting with Sam.

Her last statement came at me in slow motion, creeping into my veins languidly and then lashing at my senses like a tornado.

I blinked once, twice, and again.

Wait a second! *Did she just comment on my appearance?*

I couldn't shake the thought out of my head. I looked around to see if something had gone wrong at the venue; perhaps somebody tripped and got the tables to clatter. But nothing was out of the ordinary. Cindy and Ann were still cheerfully chatting away, and Bitul was now keenly listening to Professor Debina who was addressing the gathering from the podium.

All was very well.

The next few hours went by in a haze. I talked and laughed but also felt disoriented, losing my appetite and simply nibbling at my food.

I kept telling myself I was being silly but couldn't control the storm of emotions arising in my brain. I was lending myself to it helplessly. She surely was not commenting on my weight!

I reached my hotel well into the night and didn't sleep well.

The next day was packed with more merrymaking lined up. I avoided the full-length mirror as I got dressed. Back at the venue, I walked into the breakfast area, where Bitul came to me again, completely oblivious to the effect her comment had on me. We spent a good amount of time chatting since she was keen on learning about my practice.

I was back to normal, and by evening, I chided myself for overthinking everything. Bitul had graciously expressed respect for my work, and I was just being jealous. I promised to keep in touch, and I meant it. The evening was a riot, with the entire gang landing at the Barrel Beer Fest.

I reached New York on Tuesday morning. Nolan and Hazel were waiting for me at the door. Oh! How I had missed them. I felt like sobbing but just said a cheerful "Hi" as we hugged. I seemed to be getting all touchy… Nolan had a client meeting to attend after dropping off Hazel at kindergarten, and I had the day to myself to unwind. I'd resume work only tomorrow.

As I went about some chores, the same ugly feelings resurfaced. It was as if I had been cut open and the suppressed devils had found their way out again. They were dancing all over me. I didn't feel strong or confident but spent and weary. One part of me was astounded at this. I was at war with myself.

I had to talk to Jane.

CHAPTER 3

JANE!

SCAN FOR AUDIO CHAPTER

I first met Jane at the periphery of the Sheep Meadow in Central Park. Winter was setting in as if to rub in deeper the pain of living with a pandemic still looming large. But the human spirit was finding a way to pop its adamant head out.

I felt a surge of positivity as I jogged feeling the breeze whip at my skin. Jane was there like many other senior citizens visiting the place in the mornings. I was the only one out of place. I had reached this point earlier than my usual 7 a.m. timeline and had run up toward the meadow—not my usual route.

Jane was elegantly dressed and easygoing with an undeniable aura. She perhaps was in her late 50s, and I was immediately drawn to her enigmatic demeanor. She would laugh with the kids even though she was not part of their play and engage with people with quiet confidence. The only adjective I could think of to describe her was *stable*.

It's difficult to put into words. She appeared to exude everything that I did not. The sublime vitality around her jarred with my neurotic self. She was a little taller, with a bony structure and a well-toned body as opposed to my soft, flabby frame. I consoled myself thinking I had another 20 years to be like her.

We frequently ran into each other during my Sunday morning jogs to the park. I can proudly show off these jogs across the high line to the park as a ritual I have managed to keep alive. Talking to Jane made it all more pleasurable. I loved talking to her, even if it was about nothing in particular. She just seemed to have the answers to all my unasked questions. Catching up with her felt like a much-needed repose.

I watched as she performed yoga and took time to guide the dozens of students who gathered on the lawns eager to learn from her. It was tempting to join the group, but I was reluctant to take the initiative. I would probably not continue with it after all.

"I am here at the park every day. I teach yoga in the mornings for an hour to anyone who wants to learn," she told me. "I don't charge or ask questions." She elaborated, picking up a fallen sugar maple leaf to admire it.

A few weeks after we first met, Jane invited me to join her at the tiny coffee shop outside the park. "I love coming here alone once in a while," she said as we turned a corner and got into a narrow lane. We stopped at what was clearly someone's house for a long time. Why didn't I notice this place before? It was a quaint little place hidden behind a rich foliage of carefully manicured ferns hanging from old gray birch trees. It was much cooler here than it was just 20 feet away.

A smiling young lady opened the creaky, wooden-framed stained glass door. She looked hip and classy and was certainly a student. The aroma of freshly brewed coffee drew me in. There were just three wooden tables, all unoccupied.

"Jane," I caught myself whispering and immediately upped my volume to sound normal. "What a charming place this is!" I gushed, ogling at the minimalist designs that penetrated my nerves like a soothing balm. The coffee arrived in elegant mugs. The tiny canister of liquid palm sugar convinced me to have sweetened coffee after ages.

"I have learned to avoid sugar with a lot of effort. Managing weight is such a task," I casually said to Jane. "You only need to be wary of the hidden sugars, not the ones presented to you in these exquisite jars," she remarked, pouring herself another cup. I paused, unprepared for that observation.

"Jane, you know, when I was in high school, I had for a long time harbored a secret yearning to pass for a Parisian—sophisticated fashion, cuisine, and all of it," I told her. She laughed. "Now you don't want to be one? I am French by birth, Maya, and American in spirit; I've been here for three decades now."

"You were asking about yoga. I had pursued it for a while. My previous experience with meditation and yoga, I must admit, was not very enchanting. On the contrary, it triggered discomfort, and I am now reluctant to try again. It got too slow and boring," I blabbered away, wondering how I could be so honest with her. But I did not want to tell her that it did not appear to offer a path to weight loss, at least to me.

"I get it," said Jane serenely. "It's like trying to harness a storm. It's not easy, and eventually, when you can, you will realize that what you can do is not small."

I did not know how to carry on the conversation further because I was kind of expecting some preaching. But none came even though I showed my keenness in listening to her speak. I hoped she would try to convince me I was wrong in my understanding but no such luck. I knew she had a very sure definition of yoga, and I was missing it by miles.

Jane got me curious. I had met her only recently and found myself looking forward to another conversation even though I didn't have any particular agenda. Over the next few days, I had gotten into a kind of rumination. Every break I took, between work or at home, I would spend thinking. About what? I had no clue! Darn! I tried to brush it off, but it continued to nag me. I decided to ask Jane to be my yoga teacher. That finally seemed to settle my mind.

"Here's the deal. We are going to have the yoga sessions in your office. I'll come over once a week," she finally answered after patiently hearing me rant about lack of time.

"Jane!" I exclaimed. "The office environment is different. You may not even recognize me there!" Jane surely had no idea how the chambers functioned. That was a preposterous suggestion, I observed with empathy for her naivety. I finally felt I had an upper hand over her unassuming command.

"Maya," she said with finality, "The sessions will be at your office."

I told her I wanted to pay her for her time, and she told me her hourly rate. I charge 15 times that an hour, I thought to myself. "You will be paying a heavy price," she said as if she read my mind. "You would be sacrificing an hour, and that's a lot in terms of money." I couldn't believe I was having this conversation.

She said she'd meet me at my office on Friday evening. I did not refuse. Not because I couldn't or wanted to humor her but because I couldn't deny the authority in her tone. I owed her no obligation and could just disappear, but some faint emotion was asking me to stay put.

She was there at my office on Friday evening, sharp and on time. The ambiance of the chambers did not seem to faze her one bit.

"Well, just be seated as you are. Close your eyes and focus on your breathing. Notice the inhalation and exhalation," said Jane as she sat across the table in my office. She realized I was shifting.

"Is it difficult? Then do it with your eyes open. You don't have to face me. Look at the coffee mug and focus on your breathing. I'll keep counting for you. Stay on till I count to 10," she said helpfully, and I willingly lent myself to her instructions.

At 6 p.m., my mind began to whirl. It occurred to me that I was running behind schedule with the contract to be submitted by the day's end. I hadn't called back Bezz from P&G and Hazel needed green shoes for her skit!

"Jane, this is not working!" I blurted out. "Wrong timing perhaps," I said, looking apologetic.

"You did well for today, I think," she said with no trace of sarcasm or annoyance at having such a non-compliant student.

"But you came so far just for me." I was thoroughly ashamed of my reaction.

"I have succeeded in initiating you," she said. "Do this over and over. It will take weeks before you can reach the count of 10. I will come over again next Friday."

I had never felt so challenged. I could analyze complex legalities and play out ruthless strategies with an opponent in court, but Jane was here telling me I would not be able to breathe in and out to the count of 10, and I had no rebuttal.

Over the next few days, I tried. I tried with all sincerity. I'd forget to practice for the most part, and when I'd remember, I would not progress much. When I did not get anywhere, I began to look for resources on breathing and yoga. I called Jane, and she asked me to research like I would on the job.

"Skim through resources, sift the good advice from the bad, and draw an actionable plan." She was speaking like a law professor. I liked it. I felt like a novice again, when I was vulnerable and shaky and got away knowing someone had my back.

Jane counseling me into efficiency was a possibility, but juggling through life was my reality. The constant demands, pushbacks, and expectations I set for myself continued to be my companions. For instance, the COVID-19 lockdown last year and subsequent work-from-home juggle busted the hell out of me. Hazel and Nolan's constant presence in the background as I worked and work looming behind me on the computer screen as I turned my back to check on my house made me feel like I was being stalked the whole time and that I needed to escape from myself.

CHAPTER 4

ON A RAMPAGE ANYTIME, ANYWHERE

SCAN FOR AUDIO CHAPTER

8:00 a.m. an early morning blast

"Hey, Mae! How about going four-wheeling this Sunday? We can have a farm lunch and get back early," Nolan asked as I hurried to the porch on Wednesday morning. Midweek was always super tight, which affected my mood.

"What the hell, Nolan!" I snapped. "Is this a thing to talk about in the morning? I'll be drained by the time it's the weekend—

there is so much to do. We are no scrawny teenagers to be messing up in the slush. I have no energy." I continued angrily, barely stopping for a breath, "Can't you see I am gaining weight! You keep planning lunches without a care in the world!"

Anger spewed out of me like lava, sentences filled with accusations on how my life was going all out of my control with nobody to empathize with as Nolan continued to stare at me speechless. I heard myself, but the words wouldn't stop. I slumped on the steps as I saw Nolan's perplexed face.

"It's okay, dear. You are stressed. That's all," said Nolan, racing forward to sit next to me and give me a reassuring hug. I let the tears fall and sat there feeling both relieved at having let out the tension and repentant for having been unfair to Nolan.

"You are beating yourself up, Mae. Let's talk in the evening if you have to rush now. I promise we will find a way out," he said.

"Noli, I am so sorry. I didn't mean to blame you for the mess I am in," I said, feeling awful about the unprovoked early morning showdown.

"I think you need the four-wheeling and lunch badly—more than I do." He laughed as I rolled my eyes at him.

"Seriously Mae, you are being negative about your body and judging your life unfairly. That's why you're having these self-defeating thoughts. You really need to pause for a while and change the track of your thought process. We will not let it fester like this." The conviction in his voice acted like a balm on my throbbing head.

"Listen, I am completely with you in your desire for change but not like this! Let's find a smart way out." He gave me a pat on the cheek, and we left for work. I was getting into a vicious cycle, and it was spilling over. As I drove to work, I was overcome with a resolve to set things right.

My husband, a hardworking techie and loving family man also had long office hours and a sedentary work style. We were in the same boat; he too was not in a position to keep an active routine as much as he desired. Having said that, he did not get into a negative spiral like me. He had reconciled with the fact that opportunities for physical activity were limited now, but he would snatch them the moment a window of possibility presented itself. I was the "have it all or nothing" kind and ended up behaving like a jerk.

7:00 p.m. a run in with Zoya

"There she is!" I involuntarily jerked as I saw my neighbor Zoya returning home from her regular shopping spree. I was driving back home and badly wanted to sip on some strong coffee. "She is hiding behind a facade, presenting a sorted-out face to people, but I'm sure she is miserable when left to herself," I mumbled to myself.

"What's wrong with you, Maya?!" I chided myself, wondering why I was making snap, unprovoked judgments about people. Something like intolerance was building in me about things that were superficial and unsustainable. It was like I was craving hidden answers to construct my definition of graceful living.

"Hey, Mayz! Darling, stop!" She shrieked joyfully as she spotted my car, just as I had begun to speed up to avoid coming into her range of vision.

"Hell!" I screeched to a halt and pulled up, muttering to myself. "Hey, Zoya! Long time..."

Before I knew it, I was sipping tea in her manicured garden. She undeniably had a way of making people warm up to her. Zoya went about with her chatter and wanted me to check out all her Zara on-sale purchases. She constantly gushed over how she was on a wardrobe overhaul with her new size.

"Boy! I lost 15 lbs in just over a month. My clothes couldn't keep up." She let out an exasperated sound and waited for my eyes to pop out. By now, she was all too familiar with the reactions she invited from people. Zoya was older than me by perhaps five or some years and had recently made an image makeover her life's purpose. Well, we all crave it, I admit, but she did not believe in keeping her ambitions discreet; that was the only difference.

"I noticed that." I don't think she missed the "how the heck" in my tone.

"I'll tell you; no secrets with best friends you know!" She guffawed in all fakeness. "I got this pill online. It seems it is a well-kept secret in Oriental medicine and cost me a fortune."

"Zoya, are you sure it's okay to consume pills just like that?" I could not hold back my concern. All my attempts to enquire about its authenticity, safety, and long-term effects and my protests about marketing gimmicks sounded limp as she fiercely defended the product and her decision. I thought it would be wiser for me to give up and concede my failure in stumbling upon such treasures.

"You poor thing, look at how overworked you are," she added for that condescending effect. "I might be able to give you some self-care tips. You want me to check out something online for you dear?"

After escaping from a volley of her unsolicited advice, I entered home to find Nolan back home early and waiting for me.

"How was your day? Feeling better after beating the daylights out of me in the morning?" He grinned. When I narrated my encounter with Zoya, we agreed over a toast of wine that flaring up once in a while was better than popping unknown pills.

"I am pretty sure she is just hallucinating about losing pounds every time she notices a sale," Nolan observed.

Zoya, me, or all of us for that matter seem to be in an unending quest for elusive happiness, and we find our own quirky ways through it.

"I honestly don't understand what I can do to change my routine. I know that I need time to take care of myself but don't know how to make time for it. There's so much to do, and I am in a completely different state of mind most of the time. It is impossible to devote time and energy to myself," I admit to Nolan.

"I agree with what you are saying, dear. Let's figure something out by brainstorming and trying new ways," stated Nolan. "Just don't forget you are not alone in this. Everyone we meet is going through similar dilemmas and responding in their own ways. I am excited to see how we are going to respond. Come on, let's go for a stroll."

He had a way of putting things in perspective. I was glad that I had spoken up and even gladder that Nolan had paid attention. He was one person with whom I could be completely vulnerable.

Over the next few days, I made my notes—nope, not on the high-profile brief I was handling but on how self-neglect was creeping into my life slowly and steadily. I scribbled away in all earnestness, pages and pages of how I have been going about my routine, diet, sleep hours, moods, and overall habits. Once I was done with the writing, I sat back to read and, for the first time, saw my own patterns as if I were reading about somebody else. I found it amusing that the person in my journal had such lopsided priorities, and it was supposed to be me!

How would I judge this person? Most of all, how would I help them? If I were to get involved, I would begin by asking why.

Why do you neglect yourself?

"I do not! What makes you think so? I am only doing the things that I am supposed to do so I am successful at everything I lay my hands on." I protested, annoyed at the audacious assumption.

Going by your statement, I presume self-neglect is essential to your definition of success. Maybe you are not to be blamed completely.

"It is accepted and expected of us, and we blindly follow patterns," I retorted.

Follow-up messages from yesterday's client meeting flooded my inbox. I decided not to open them right away because I wanted to clock in my workout. I was gradually beginning to enjoy the high that came over me post-workout. It was a pity that I had gotten into the habit of getting sloshed with caffeine to overcome my lethargy and low moods. Now, I would have coffee when I wanted to not because I had to.

Jane had left me a card in which she wrote a few notes on how I could take my first steps to chair yoga, something that would take less than five minutes to read. She asked me to use them over the next few weeks.

I decided to begin practice in the morning. I got up earlier than usual and got myself a chair next to the window. I stared into the morning sky and got lost in my thoughts. The haze signified the arrival of winter, and it was already becoming unbearable to anticipate a cheerful morning. The silence of the mornings felt unfamiliar. It had been years since I woke up and didn't rush. This morning was honestly looking bizarre. The warm blanket was irresistibly inviting, and nothing appeared more divine or purposeful than being able to slip under it. I came out of my reverie when Jane's note slipped off my hands. I need to do the exercises; I chide myself and read through them. I was a bit nervous after that breathing-to-the-count-of-10 disaster in the office.

There were two warm-up instructions and two yoga poses: the mountain and tree pose. I can do this much today. Jane shouldn't have underestimated me. At least 10 poses in four weeks would have been a fair pace, not two.

I did the warm-ups, and it felt good to move my joints and stretch after a long time. I was an accomplished volleyball player in high school and felt nostalgic. Alright, the next one. I looked into the notes and read through both. The mountain pose looked easy. I sat upright with complete awareness of my body and closed my eyes.

That's better! I complimented myself. Now pay attention to breathing. Inhale, hold, exhale, repeat… inhale, hold, exhale, repeat… I heard the alarm go off and footsteps approaching. "Good morning, Maya," Nolan's tone was cautious. "You alright?"

"Oh, yes, I am doing some exercises!"

"You're sure?" he asked, looking at me sitting on the chair.

I laughed. "Sure, sure! Now make us some coffee." I hadn't told him about my yoga lessons yet, my bad!

I got back in position and closed my eyes

The neighbor's dog barked.

Oh, I needed to tell Gerard about the copyright clause.

Hazel has not been eating her cereal, so it's pancakes today, darn!

I have an appointment with the hairdresser at 6…

The purposeful thoughts gushed in viciously as I was sitting on the chair seemingly without any particular goal. I jumped up. "Nolan, is the coffee ready?" I rushed out of the room in desperation.

5:00 p.m. a taste of being with myself

"Perfect! Be prepared for more such experiences. Your mind and body will resist with all their might." I had given up on being startled by Jane's responses by now.

"I will ask you to stay with the experiences and lend yourself to the chair again and again. Just know that you are nourishing yourself. "That was how she concluded our 40-second phone conversation.

It dawned on me that the idea of being with myself was alien to me. I could spend a long time thinking of something or working on something. However, just being, without any apparent purpose, only baffled me. I instinctively knew I was missing something, but I was clueless. Jane would surely help me.

9:00 a.m. much ado about time

My Sunday morning jog was all I had managed to sustain in all these years in the name of exercise. "Tell me," she asked when I met her on Sunday, "why did you pick the mountain pose over the tree one to begin?"

"It was the easier of the two," I said. But I felt unsure when I turned to look at her.

"Both are difficult ones, but the mountain pose is really difficult. It is a fundamental pose. While you can begin with poses having body movement, you can also get back to them if they are tough to sustain. They'll help you control your thoughts because your mind will focus on the movements."

"I don't quite understand."

"Look, the mind seemingly goes haywire with a zillion thoughts, but it can only think one thought at a time. There are many quick-succession single thoughts; use that limitation to your advantage, like you use loopholes to strengthen your case," she elaborated.

I have numerous stories about my trials at working out. I have bought gym memberships a dozen times and abandoned them. I have had to apologize to my trainer for asking him to keep postponing our visits. I have been too tired to wake up extra early to exercise and wanted to spend every minute possible with Hazel—she is growing up so fast.

"Chair yoga will work well for you since that is where you spend most of your time. You are not going to be able to carry a yoga mat around, let alone a whole gym. As long as you and the chair are there, yoga is a possibility," stated Jane.

"I am not implying that you should be embarrassed about having a desk job. Sitting is not as harmful as it is made out to be, so do not feel guilty. Wrong beliefs can be self-sabotaging."

"Moreover, your frame of mind will be different, or your clothes and hair will get disheveled to the dismay of your team; we will address that too." She was savage. That was exactly what I was preparing to tell her.

"There is a difference between thinking you have no time and having no time."

"Does that mean I am not being honest?"

"Yes, but not deliberately, so you will not be accused of lying," she smiled.

"Now, your clothes. You need to wear a perfectly ironed business suit to a meeting or on a court hearing day. Can we think of fabric and design options for most days that provide scope for stretching and don't compromise on your style and authority? Being forced to relook at a carefully put-together wardrobe can be annoying but consider the trade-off and make a choice. Do not shut down possibilities."

"I had a boss whom people would make fun of behind his back. He would stretch and twist and turn during business discussions and embarrass people. I don't want to look funny—that's not me!"

"You already know the repercussions, so you won't do it during conversations. That excuse is already out! Where do you sit when you spend time with Hazel in the evenings?"

"I relax on the couch."

"Where does she sit?"

"She sits on the carpet with her toys. Well, she sits wherever she likes; the floor gives her more freedom though."

As I spoke, I could see what she was getting at. "You want me to get on the floor with her?" I grinned. "Were you ever trained to be a lawyer?" I asked seriously.

"Why?" She laughed.

"You ask the right questions, and your rebuttals are sophisticated."

"Ah! My medical students think I'm a doctor, and the dancers think I am a dancer," she stated plainly. "What they don't realize is that they need to use their intellectual training to work for themselves first. Maya the lawyer needs to be her most important client; Marco the teacher, his most important student; and Jae the sales manager, her most valuable customer."

CHAPTER 5

REIGNING IN, FINALLY!

SCAN FOR AUDIO CHAPTER

5:30 p.m. I'll never *want* to work out

Perhaps for the fiftieth time, I told Jane that I didn't have time or energy for fitness. I would go into autopilot mode, complaining whenever I met her.

"It is a story you have internalized," she stated simply. "You are blaming your life situations for hindering self-care. And then, when you start taking care of your fitness, you start blaming it for affecting your work and family. Take a step back and think, Maya; aren't you getting into a loop of self-defeat?"

"True, but I can't see a way out," I lamented unabashedly.

"Let's see how you can approach your dilemmas differently. You are a lawyer and need to work for 12 to 14 hours at the desk. Is that a crime? No. But you feel guilty about it." I started to interrupt, but she continued. "Stay with me on this, dear."

I nodded, keen on understanding a different perspective.

"Have you seen any creature in nature prancing around without purpose… birds fly only when they have to, your pet moves only when it needs to, apes are more sedentary than humans, and hunter-gatherers no doubt work hard for around five to six hours a day, but the rest of the time, they sit. Our ancestors from simpler times also sat when they were not working."

"You are suggesting that having a desk job is not a hindrance, so to speak, and that it's okay. But what about the lethargy you feel post spending so much sedentary time? In all the examples you mentioned, each creature exerts themselves physically while they work, even if only for a limited time. Sedentary work cuts out physical exertion." My argument seemed very sound to me. I hoped Jane could convince me otherwise.

"Yes, agreed. There is no denying that we are becoming a chair-dependent society, and we need to know the consequences. However, we are made to feel guilty about our sitting jobs and this guilt further feeds our attitude toward exercising. Therein lies the root of the problem. We wonder why we don't feel like going for a walk or to the gym. The thing is it is not possible to want to exert ourselves until our brain is convinced of the benefits."

I slowly began to get what she was arriving at.

"The brain doesn't see sense in unnecessary physical exertion. The body will function perfectly well without voluntary functions such as exercise."

"Hmm, I see your point about the body not finding it natural to exercise, but how does this knowledge help me?"

"It helps because you're aware that choosing to work out and eat healthy food is as deliberate a process as getting up in the morning and showing up for work."

"You mean to say, I will never get to a point where I will feel like doing exercises?"

"You will not," she smiled, "unless you decide it is beneficial for you, and then get it to set in as a habit like any other."

Jane could see that I was finally starting to get it. She continued, "Very much like how money, identity, happiness, purpose, and the like are the motivating factors in your career, your present and future well-being should be motivators for taking care of yourself. What I am pointing out is that there needs to be deliberate planning and effort. There is no default exercising mode one can achieve."

"We all need assistance and must seek help to learn how to use our bodies for activity. Physical activity is inherently simple; we shouldn't complicate it."

Being of Spanish-American descent, I had only recently discovered that "Maya" meant "illusion" in Sanskrit. So, being the disillusioned person that I turned out to be, I was dis-maya-ed. But I was also beginning to see a way out!

"Wow," was all I could say as the apple cart of my misconceptions overturned in slow motion.

MY PRACTICE

After some trials, errors, and reworkings, I finally managed to set aside about 15 minutes for myself every morning. I came up with this wicked-looking plan of not allowing myself to go to the kitchen for my hot cup of coffee without first sitting on the yoga chair. After all, I had to be my most important client!

I promised to begin with the understanding that yoga was more about the mind and that the body would follow. I had to recondition my mind to stop looking at it as a bunch of impossible poses, and that would take some effort. I reminded myself that the purpose of performing chair yoga at home was to successfully replicate it during work hours.

I had to document the goings-on in my head and body if I were to keep my case strong. So here I go…

6:00 a.m. breathe in, pose out

I sat by the window and began by observing my breath, "I am breathing in….and…I am breathing out." Thoughts would start flooding in, and I was not to resist them or get attached to them. I had to bring my attention back to breathing and give my mind useful work.

Being aware of the present sounds, smells, and sensations is a good thing because we miss tangible happenings when we are lost in thought. I stopped in about five minutes when the resistance began to get stronger. The elephant had to be trained gently and over time.

Now for some body movement: I assumed the mountain pose and took my time, paying attention to my body. I had to train myself to begin to feel its sensations, and that would come in a few days. For now, feeling my feet on the ground, the chair touching my body, the shifting of my hips as I struggled to sit still, my mind trying to run in all directions, and the process of watching myself would suffice. Gradually, my breathing began to synchronize, and I saw the purpose in the pose because I was paying attention to one part of the body at a time.

This is my chance to get aligned with the idea of yoga. A person like me who had not sat on a chair except when doing something, dreaming away, or brooding over something had no clue what it meant to sit without thought.

Sitting on a chair with your spine erect, feet grounded on the floor, hands on your thighs, and eyes closed to bring awareness to the breath, body, and mind is nothing like your everyday sitting. What baffled me was the counter-intuitiveness of it all. Here I was, wanting to bring about a change in my lifestyle and take significant path-breaking steps to weight loss, but I was being ushered into "inaction."

I had to do quite a bit of reading, observing, and reflecting before I began my own practice. I realized I was dealing with a monster in this greatly deceptive calmness of a pose. I was to discover the power of silence.

Getting into action and being a go-getter is who I am, and I was setting myself up to go against it. Man! This is something of a challenge. I was afraid of the consequences of venturing into this unknown possibility and found myself wanting to feel safe in the familiar.

"Resist getting pulled away into the past or future. You will realize there is a present, perhaps for the first time in your life," Jane would remind me.

"You will want to revisit old memories and end up getting stuck in the same emotions over and over or wondering about the future and attaching emotions tied to the past. Isn't it inefficient, Maya?"

"Hmmm, I need to give it some thought; I haven't looked at it that way ever," I loved repeating these conversations with Jane because I was convinced I was missing something here.

The mountain pose, or *Tadasana*, is the base pose that one needs to master. It teaches us to center ourselves in mind and body against the tendency to be scattered. It is the one pose that will help us move to any other pose in yoga.

I like to call it the skeleton of yoga, without which every other stance is a meaningless wobbly mass of flesh. On the outside, it looks motionless, but the body is awakening every inch of itself with some parts flexing and others relaxing. As I went deeper into practice, my mind started recognizing the sensations better.

My first experience with the pose was on the first day Jane had trudged into my office. When I wept on her shoulders later telling her how impossible it felt, she asked me to join her group session at Central Park on Sundays. She took me under her wings, and we practiced amid the soothing breeze, fresh grass, and fragrant flora. I felt reassured watching my fellow practitioners.

Back on the chair next dawn! I congratulated myself on my first successful chair yoga day in the office. I moved my body more frequently and at every opportunity now. I began with the warm-ups and visualized myself bending and stretching on my chair during work. It was possible, and I was happy that my attitude had started changing.

Simply raising our hands can set off a train of incorrect body part sequencing and undermine the purpose of the pose. I discovered this when I proudly declared to Jane that I could do the raised hands pose without guidance—it looked like a no-brainer.

When I showed her, she told me that my tailbone, ribcage, and neck would go for a toss if I continued doing what I was doing. Skimming over instructions and taking things at face value would compromise my practice and take me to a dead end very soon.

Guys! Please begin your journey with a worthy teacher.

9:00 a.m. a little heart-to-heart

"It uplifts you from fatigue. On a psychological level, it stimulates your ability to communicate and express your feelings and thoughts. During your practice aim to find a sense of release. On a physiological level, it strengthens your hands and spine, preparing them for more weight-bearing poses," she explained.

I felt the urge to try out one more pose and went for the tree pose. It involved lifting your right leg, spreading your arms, and keeping your posture straight with your hands stretched up—oh my! When I tried it, I realized my body had lost its flexibility over the years. I made a mental note of every ache and discomfort and began to appreciate what bringing awareness to the body does—it starts talking to you! I would have to listen more from now on.

My first attempt at the tree pose made me aware of how I couldn't balance my body well enough. A few days of practice brought me a sense of balance and grace; I could finally stay stable on one leg. It's not difficult, just that our abilities are buried under layers of idiosyncrasies.

I noticed how my lower body held strong while my upper body worked into an elaborate stretch. Jane had asked me to watch out for the right combination of stretch and strength and eventually learn to focus on the anatomy of yoga to derive deeper benefits. I tried to get a sense of what she said, but I knew I had a long way to go. I am just about grazing the first layer of yoga.

The allotted fifteen minutes were up; I sprang up to begin my day!

"Morning, darling!" This time Meryl was caught by surprise at my easy tone. Her face lit up. Moods can be contagious, and perhaps for the first time, I felt the power of choice.

As I rushed in and out of meetings and research during the day, I found moments to return to the mountain pose. It brought the feeling of "resetting" every single time.

When I got back home in the evening, I was not as grouchy as I had gotten used to being. I readily sat down on the carpet with a fruit platter to spend those precious moments with my child. She was pleased; I was more so. I got moving along with her. I began paying attention to my body and observed that my quadriceps, core muscles, hamstrings, and hip flexors were put to work when sitting, squatting, twisting, and turning on the floor. I finally began to appreciate yoga's stretching and strengthening qualities.

I needed to be specific in my questions. Vague questions got me vague solutions. Let me try. "Can we do some yoga now?" I would ask myself. *No, not in the mood*, came the reply.

"What is stopping me from doing one pose of chair yoga just now?" I asked. *Just one is doable.*

The cat-cow pose was a clear winner. It was nonintrusive because I could do it even when I was preoccupied with work. My work spread over hours, and the expanding and contracting movement of the pose got my blood circulating better. Moving the spine in a rhythm and connecting to the breath helped me become conscious of the anxieties building up and allowed me to detach from them. I was becoming aware of my posture and checking those inadvertent slouches long after I returned to work mode.

CHAPTER 6

STUMBLING UPON SURPRISES

SCAN FOR AUDIO CHAPTER

January: Onward and upward—are we there yet?

It was not yet a "... and I lived happily ever after" story. A few months into staying consistent in my pursuits was getting me on track, but staying consistent still required a lot of effort.

I expressed my concerns about this to Jane: "I have been practicing yoga for some time now, Jane. But honestly, I still get the feeling that there is nothing significant happening in terms of visible results. I feel more in control of myself, even more poised, but nothing seems to have changed on the outside. By now, I know my physical limitations, I can feel vague sensations due to all the movement, and I am better at recognizing good pain and bad. But I am still unsure of having the motivation to carry on because I can't see weight loss."

She didn't protest. "It's tough to be alone with yourself. The body movements by themselves are only aiding the process of self-discovery. You shouldn't begin with more than 10 minutes of yoga practice."

If she had meant to challenge me with that statement, she had succeeded. "That can't be true," I argued. "It's just that there is no action." I heard how naive I sounded and continued. "It gets too difficult and overwhelming at times, Jane. It is like having another thing added to my already hectic life."

"Your worries are coming from a place of anxiety, so it is all the more important to simplify things. Trust the process, Maya. Yoga will help you remove mental and physical blocks. Right now, there is constant friction because you are being pulled in different directions. You find the need to be on high alert in all the roles, which is taxing. Yoga is all about spending time with yourself and gradually knowing yourself."

"I think I'll take it one day at a time. Thanks, Jane." The fog in my mind has cleared up a little now.

I decided to keep notes this time (after all, I was on an important case), notes on my understanding of the actions I needed to take to put my life in order. I felt super good that I was gradually keeping my morning appointment with myself. I was also glad to be getting familiar with the poses and deeper into practice.

With time, I got a fair idea of what my body could do and where it needed improvement. I keenly followed the hip-opening poses and spine-relaxing twists and turns with extremely gentle movements to get the flow. A simple pose or exercise sometimes took weeks to achieve. The seemingly small daily gains started to stack up. Some days were exhausting and discouraging no doubt, but I could already feel a shift in my attitude and a lift in my energy.

Standing on one leg without wobbling would look impossible on some days. I would be overcome with lethargy at the thought of moving my hands and legs on other days. Sometimes, I'd wonder if I could learn a certain pose in a month. But there was no deadline to meet; I only had to focus on the form.

Finding the balance between making an effort and surrendering came with experience. I would eventually get to the benefits of the pose, but not before I did my part in allowing my body to open up. I soon began to notice the dull aches, the feelings coming from a place of fear, as I began spending time with myself.

The journey was not smooth by any means. Feelings of self-doubt and lethargy would keep crawling in. But this time instead of giving up without realizing, I was becoming strongly aware of negative feelings and taking the initiative to talk to Jane about them. Something was different about my inaction as well…

ON WHY I HAVE BEEN RELUCTANT TO DO YOGA

I was making assumptions for a very long period. Instead of trying to learn yoga, I was relying on informal comments and perceptions I gathered from all kinds of sources. I should have been aware that using the hearsay approach in legal research would be unacceptable; no one could use second-hand information to be successful in their line of work. When I thought of yoga, I imagined people with incredibly flexible bodies that appeared to have bendy bones, and my immediate conclusion was—it's not for me!

With a few days of open-minded observations, I realized that yoga's highly adaptable approach made it incredibly suitable for a novice like me or anyone with medical conditions, the young and old, and the fit and not so fit. Inspirational Instagram yoga posts did not help me at this point. The mind-blowing poses displayed there made me feel more inadequate than inspired.

On Saturday morning, I got carried away and pushed myself. I was left with a sprain and unable to practice yoga for the week that followed. The fear of pain crept into me, and the sight of the chair reminded me of it. It was a pathetic situation, and I needed a way out.

"You focused on the results and lost awareness of the process; otherwise, you would have heard when your neck was asking you to stop," said Jane when I told her about the injury.

Ah! I should have realized. This also led me to think about what imitation does. While feeling inspired by others' success stories, I missed an important point about silent evidence.

That silent evidence was not visible. Injured people visiting a physiotherapist didn't go about posting their stories for all to see. Even if some brave soul posted one, it wouldn't get as many views. I was focusing on the success stories, not realizing that many of us trying to push possibilities end up with injuries that prevent us from doing anything at all.

In his unconventional book, "The Black Swan," Nassim Nicholas Taleb (2017) shares an interesting theory about how we determine what leads us to success

He speaks on how we base our conclusions on success stories that are visible, whereas the graveyard bears the silent evidence of people who have failed despite displaying the same attributes as the successful. We get taken over by the survivorship bias, where we focus on what worked and overlook what did not work.

I needed to watch my actions.

ON ACTIVITY (SURPRISE, SURPRISE!)

Wanting to move your body when you don't have to is akin to me trying to argue a case in an empty courtroom. There would just be no motivation. My grand plans of drawing out time for some physical activity would be put on the back burner when the demands of the day would present themselves, and I would be left feeling bad about it after the day passed. There is, however, a twist in the tale.

From an evolutionary standpoint, our brains think it is abnormal to exert the body when there is no immediate need or threat. Daniel E. Liberman (2020), in busting many cultural and urban myths, points out the fallacies of our popular understanding of exercise.

In pre-industrialized societies, our ancestors were active enough to feed, protect, and entertain themselves but never performed physical activities to maintain health. This need came in very recently when we began to sit on chairs for monthly paychecks. Our brain still wonders why we have to move when we don't have to—it considers it harassment.

Turns out, my body is doing a lot of work even in its seemingly inactive state. It will use up calories for its functioning based on what I put in and store the excess, thus making it my responsibility to watch what I put in. I will have to decide to work out every single time I do so—it has to be a conscious, well-planned decision.

No default mental or physical setting will make me feel like exercising. Every single time I pick up my training shoes or get on the mat, I should thank myself for making time for it. Moreover, one successful day does not mean another; you are essentially fighting a deep-rooted instinct to conserve energy.

This knowledge knocked the entire burden of guilt out of my story. Imagine how we beat ourselves up for not setting aside time and finding reasons to indulge in self-pity. This stems from a strong belief that we are supposed to "want" to exercise because not doing so means we are lazy or irresponsible. I see a lot of passionate people around making me feel that we are born to exercise.

With this realization, I felt like an alleged criminal being honorably cleared of all charges. I could now design my days without blaming myself. I wish I had a magic wand to banish the strongly conditioned guilt out of my life.

The one challenge I could see in the coming days was trying to discern what would work for me. We live in times where exercise, though inherently free, is a multi-billion-dollar industry, and sifting the wheat from the chaff would not be child's play. Making us feel like fancy workouts are the only way to live longer and healthier has an ulterior motive, which adds to the confusion. I needed to know about what would help me exercise, not things that made it complicated. Imagine failing to do what I wanted to because of analysis paralysis.

ON DESIGNING MY DAYS

As I spent more time practicing yoga, I realized that I tended to deprioritize my needs. The first thing to fly out of the window when the reality of the day kicked in was me-time.

How could I design my days with this mental blueprint? For me, me-time was like an indulgence kept in the realm of wishful thinking. But that's how everyone works, right? I have not seen many role models around me do otherwise.

My family values, religion, society, and education did not endorse me-time loud and clear; it's simply not natural. But they did have terms to describe a person who acknowledged their own needs—selfish, self-centered, egoistic, and anti-social.

Children and rebellious teenagers are tolerated for such behavior, although everyone waits for them to grow up. Assertiveness is so vital but is not a quality taught to us. We imbibe social and belief barriers to remain passive and go with the flow.

I always allowed my inner critic to bulldoze my intentions of changing by convincing me that I had to "save" my energy for "important stuff." I had to stop making exercise a source of anxiety and instead make it easy and fun.

I successfully rid myself of guilt but wondered whether I could banish fear as well. I was fascinated with the idea of removing all negative connotations of exercising so that it could become a truly blissful activity.

Based on Jane's recommendation from the other day, I decided to take another look at some of our deeply entrenched beliefs. We carry them all the time without a second thought; they're truly automatic.

It appears fashionable in the industrialized world to believe that city dwellers are "artificial" beings while forest dwellers are "authentic" ones. We also live in fear that our luxuries are out to kill us. Observing forest dwellers, however, reveals that they spend lots of time relaxing once the day's survival needs are met. They don't eat junk food, but they do while away their time.

I dealt with a highly sensitive case last week and spent every iota of my time and energy on the nuances of the case. It was hours and hours of intense work with many nasty surprises. Only after we waded through it did I realize that I had missed working out for a whole week. I had done none of the poses or breathing exercises that could have helped me cope with the stress and respond better to the situation.

I was disheartened. This was a setback because I was somehow convinced that I could only exercise when I had the luxury of time. I needed to spend enough time developing an exercise routine during normal days to internalize it as a process that would work for me during stressful times too.

I found my little success in another situation that followed. A few weeks later, Hazel was down with a nasty intestinal infection that led to a week's hospitalization. It was a distressing time for Nolan and me. We had to be at multiple important places while making sure Hazel came out safe and well from the ordeal.

I discovered that I could practice yoga and breathwork in little increments to truly experience their benefits. I was managing without losing it and acutely aware of how my mental processes were altering.

As I sat in the hospital chair watching Hazel, frail but fighting back, I would spend a few hours on the laptop catching up on work and getting my yoga poses going. I would take short walks in the ward corridors and find breathing exercises particularly relaxing. The animated feeling of stress was shaken up every time I lent myself to some physical activity. My moods would significantly alter for the better, and I would feel ready to cope with any situation.

I AM SHOWING PROGRESS

I used to find all yoga instructions similar and repetitive. I recognized my naivety only when I started experiencing each pose for myself. My body would move according to its tendencies, and I would feel a loss of control over the movements. I realized that my default movements were a concoction of faulty habits combined with ignorance of how muscles needed to activate and knowledge of how joints behaved.

I was keen on learning something new this morning that I could apply during work hours. The aches and pains and lack of stamina I felt while doing chair yoga directly affected my nutritional deficiencies. I had to watch my food intake if I wanted to sustain myself.

Time to close off the loopholes in my lawsuit!

Now that I was getting friendlier with my body, I had another brain wave in the morning. I asked Jane to teach me both the floor and chair variations of the poses. I could practice floor yoga at home and chair yoga at work!

I repeated the breathing exercise, mountain pose, and tree pose. It was getting better, and so were my listening-to-my-body capabilities. I tried the raised hand poses and their variations, which gave me the nicest side stretches. They felt like an instant upper body massage with the spine lengthening and ribcage relaxation filling me with vigor. I soon discovered their ability to help me focus on my job too!

Over the next few weeks, I began to get into the groove. It was about feeling one with yourself—trust me, it is not easy. We are very happy to be scattered, contradictory creatures of habit.

Developing the right mindset while performing the poses was more difficult than performing the poses. I had to keep reminding myself to get in the appropriate state of mind. Trying to maintain proper posture would often cause me to lose focus and fail to pay attention. I had to persevere because this needed a lot of conditioning. Being respectful and compassionate to yourself was more challenging than I thought.

I needed to break down the problem into simpler bits and be kinder to myself. To master the pose—stay in the position for a long duration, I needed to stretch my forearms and ribs, open up my hips, get my inner thighs used to the movement, and work on strengthening my core. I had to look for the precursor *asanas* (poses)—the simple ones that would help me twist, stretch, and sustain—to finally reach that level. I looked at my yoga notes and discovered a treasure trove to choose from.

I found the tree pose and its variations easy today. Keeping my arms high up with one leg stretched was relaxing as my spinal cord began to feel less stiff. It helped me get over the wobbling I experienced initially. I was beginning to build better balance.

The hands-to-toe pose was also a revealing experience. I only need to bend and touch the toes of my extended right leg. In about eight seconds, I could feel the stretch on my entire spinal cord, the nerves of my arm, and my hamstring. My neck was straining, and I could no longer hold the position. My belly flab was making things worse. I couldn't bend on the left side well.

With Jane's help, I found some workarounds. I began to look for opportunities to loosen up my hamstrings at home, in the park, and pretty much wherever I went. Opportunities were everywhere if you looked for them. I would stretch my legs on the chair seat at home, the high coffee table while standing, or the landscaping in the garden or bend while waiting for the kettle to boil.

CHAPTER 7

ARE WE AFRAID OF CHANGE?

SCAN FOR AUDIO CHAPTER

4:00 p.m. we're not in this alone

"I do not aspire to be a model. I have a demanding schedule, managing home and work, which calls for a lot of physical activity in any case."

Clearly, my colleague Julia did not see anything wrong with not having a thought-out fitness plan. It got me thinking about how we all tend to leave so much to chance but are not happy with the consequences.

Julia had two school-going kids aged eight and twelve. We were all used to her frantic instructions to her kids and hubby on the phone at least a dozen times a day.

"Now that you mention it, Maya," she continued as an afterthought. "I know it's only a matter of time before I have trouble in my relationship with the kids or John. I am already at my wit's end." She was welling up.

"I am sorry I got you overwhelmed. Come on, let's get some coffee."

"Oh, no. It's okay. I think it's important to talk about these things," she continued. "I feel like I've messed up everything and can't enjoy work or home," she confessed as we strolled down the slushy footpath. The morning rain had a calming effect on the city and perhaps got many of us in a reflective mood today.

"I am distracted whenever John wants to spend time with me. I feel so inadequate… and have become a to-do list vending machine of sorts. I need to do something about it before all hell breaks loose." She seemed to be doing some serious calculations in her head.

"You know something, Maya. My mother worked hard to bring up four kids single-handedly. But she made it look easy! Despite having achieved so much in my career and having a stable family, I feel I am nowhere close to being as successful as she was. I lack the fulfillment she can boast of. Imagine my kids remembering me as someone who ran about like a headless chicken." I had to admit she had a point.

I find myself thinking Julia should be doing this and Julia should be doing that… but what about me? I am no different from her. I don't understand what it is that I want from life.

I don't want to face my fears or reevaluate my definition of success and happiness. Perhaps it's high time I dared to look at my authentic self.

I realized the need for tools to discern relevant information from the various theories about exercise, diet, and lifestyle and build the discipline to derive the benefits and become more efficient in everything I do.

The way forward now was to dissect the complex into chewable bits and move ahead in good faith. Learning from mistakes, training to be patient, and changing my beliefs had to be an integral part of the process, while self-compassion needed to be the underlying constant.

I began by noting my mental barriers one by one and trying to find a way out of each of them. I looked at them objectively, which helped me come up with solutions. Otherwise, it would always end up in self-pity or self-loathing.

THE ELEPHANT AND THE RIDER

I want to change my habits. I am, no doubt, ambitious about getting into shape. I don't always have to be told what needs to be done. Now if only I could figure out why I don't do what needs to be done...

I needed to check if I was setting myself up for changes in my behavior. I knew it was not about willpower but something more—what was it?

Jonathan Haidt (2006) talks about 10 great ideas. One of them beautifully explains why self-improvement is so difficult. We continue to do what we know is terrible for us despite knowing the consequences.

Imagine your brain comprising two parts: the reasoning part is the rider and the emotional part is the larger elephant. The rider decides that regular workouts are good for you but can do nothing much when the elephant says it's too cozy under the blanket to be getting up early for that.

The solution is not confrontation because the tiny rider will be no match but gradual training, coaxing, and distraction so the elephant will follow the rider's instructions. This means that using only willpower won't do—you must be strategic—something like bundling a new habit with an old one. Perhaps moving your body whilst on a chair?

MY RELATIONSHIP WITH FOOD

8:00 p.m. let's get this bread!

Jane had left me a message. It read, "Can I ask you to look up resources on nutrition if you are keen? I will be happy to get into a conversation about food."

Is she putting me on a treasure hunt? I mused. The mention, however, triggered a lot of questions about my habits. I suspected it would not be an easy conversation. I frankly never had a serious dialogue on why I ate what I ate.

I decided to track my eating. I picked up patterns over the years: eating what was remaining on Hazel's plate, finishing up cookies she was no longer interested in, and indulging in packaged "healthy" and "unhealthy" snacks as I waited in the parking lot.

I was carrying forward a lot of food preferences out of sheer habit. Every other client meeting was at lunchtime with food being ordered in to get the long discussions going. Watching what I ate was the last thing that crossed my mind. I would begin with a sugarless cup of coffee, but the following helpings were taken when I was mentally drained, which justified the sugar.

I needed to clean up my act, but it was not easy. One part of me would resist such good intentions with all its might. It was the elephant and the rider at play. I had to choose simple steps before gently prodding the elephant without letting it know.

I promptly fixed an appointment with the lab for some bloodwork, which pointed to vitamin and iron deficiencies. I then met with my doctor and followed up on the supplements they recommended to address the deficiencies.

"The pills will help you make up for deficiencies until you modify your diet to get them from your food," she said.

I sat down to make notes on what I ate in a day. Wholesome, nutritious foods were far and few. The rest of the page had processed food, refined carbs, hidden sugar and salt, coffee, and more coffee. My intake of micronutrients and complex carbohydrates was being compromised every day. But how did I end up this way? The answer turned out to be simple: accessibility. Processed food is easily available, storable, and portable.

I had a new problem. I couldn't lay my hands on fresh, wholesome food. Changing cooking patterns built over the years seemed like an insurmountable task. Every time I tried changes, it would last only a few days. Then, I would reset to default mode without even realizing it.

I sought out exotic solutions before realizing that fear is a highly marketable commodity. To put healthy food on the table, I didn't have to scour the market for exorbitantly priced "organic, pesticide-free, grass-fed, non-GMO... the works." I kept an eye out for fresh, in-season food and looked up simple traditional recipes.

9:00 a.m. off to the farmer's market

"Do little things one step at a time," Jane emphasized. "Write down every time you score a small victory so that you see it with your eyes again and again."

Jane put it this way: "We have grown up in an industrialized society raring to go with youthful energy, showing the world how innovation can lead to prosperity. In the process of building a new world, the meaning of food also began to change. To become more efficient, we began to find ways of making food storable, transportable, and flexible. Many things picked up fresh from the farmer, cooked, and promptly eaten were replaced with things that could be preserved, stored, and eaten at will. It was a trade-off we had reconciled to."

So today, a bowl of freshly baked sweet potatoes would be easily substituted with a packet of crisps, and life would go on, rather efficiently, because we would still have time to do useful stuff. What we failed to realize was that, in the long term, there can be no success in life if wellness is not a prominent ingredient.

"The problem is in the process; by default, our environments set us up to be undernourished and overweight. To reclaim our health, we now need to swim against the tide. Nothing around will allow for it because we have built our lifestyle to synchronize with rushed living. It would appear rather silly to be otherwise. See for yourself: Every time you reach out to consume anything, bring your attention to its source. Make a mental note of whether it is processed or straight off the farm. It is time to bend the curve, one choice at a time!" she reflected.

I looked at my notes and decided I couldn't become a saint overnight! I needed to direct my anger somewhere. I targeted it on those sneaky extras on my plate and in my cup—might as well take it out on something that will work to my advantage. What's life without some revenge?

"I had no idea we had a weekend market five miles away, Nolan. Hazel's teacher had mentioned they were planning to take the children for a visit."

"Yeah, somebody had mentioned it when we moved here. But the supermarket is convenient for us, right? Just run across and pick up something fresh, no hassle," said Nolan, still checking his accounts. "I think we should go Saturday morning with Hazel," I insisted, and we went.

Walking through the different trails of the fresh market with its burst of colors and whiffs of fresh produce was a revelation. The smell of mud, the chaos, and the rustic ambiance was a far cry from the sight of plastic-wrapped produce in the silent, air-conditioned, sanitized spaces of the supermarket.

My first response was a deep sense of guilt for denying ourselves, and particularly our growing child, the stimulus of nature—the real world. Hazel was initially stupefied. Gradually, she relaxed and rather enjoyed the feast of the senses. It simply seemed the right place to be.

"We will go every week from now on. Gosh! I had even forgotten certain vegetables existed," declared Nolan as we organized the veggies and fruits in the refrigerator and stocked batches of minced meatballs in the freezer. I loved the idea of prepping multiple meals.

My mind gushed with ideas of cooking dishes I had only eaten at grandma's place when I was a kid. I very much wanted Hazel to also have good memories of bonding and learning to share and care. I realized today that all this happens through the medium of food. Take away the food factor, and we lose out on all the dynamics.

I resorted to the usual pancake and syrup or egg and bread formula a few times, and I would pay the price by going through the painful act of throwing rotting vegetables out and learning my lesson.

4:30 p.m. there's more to food than just eating

Today, I mulled over how I should approach my relationship with food. My appetite depended on my current emotional frame. I ate less when I was in a hurry and ate fast when I had an appointment. The quantity would depend on the occasion. I ate more in the company of friends, during festivities, and at family get-togethers and skimped during business meals.

But that is the beauty of food: It is contextual, emotional, cultural, social, and deeply personal. It is much more than an assortment of nutrients. I had to accept that appetite varies, and resistance should be directed correctly. If Hazel keeps a piece of cake for Mamma, I should enjoy eating it with her and not let go of that magical moment due to guilt about sugar. I should rather be mindful of the hidden sugar in the office coffee break cookies.

"Fast food restaurants are easier to locate than fresh markets and convenience food is so much cheaper than whipping up a wholesome meal. Why are we surprised at the way we are shaping up?" Meryl observed as we munched on a snack last evening, with me going on about how unhealthy the popcorn chicken was. Both of us had to work late to finish vetting documents for a cranky client.

Meryl pulled out an apple from her bag along with a teeny pocketknife.

"That's cool. Do you always have fruits in stock?"

"I grab a fruit along with my car keys in the mornings. It's kind of a pair up." She grinned."That way I won't forget."

"You are quite thoughtful for your age I must say."

Meryl smiled, but I noticed a streak of despondency in her face as we hurried with work. I must get to know her better.

NOTES ON MY LIFESTYLE

9:00 p.m. what the missing dishwasher taught me

There's no point talking about fitness when you have no empathy for yourself! In the past, Nolan's willingness to help would not reach me because I would block it out with self-apathy.

Today, I lost it when I saw there was no dishwasher powder in the cupboard."How could I forget to put it on the shopping list?" I whined. But before my thoughts could cascade into a trip of self-criticism, I reined them in. Washing dishes at the sink with Nolan and catching up on some gossip was not a bad idea after all!

I needed to set myself up for success. Knowing that I would resist, I had to nudge myself every single day to do a little bit for myself. The little notes I made on new workouts and the process of trial and error seemed to be adding up to something. I was beginning to accept that managing weight and building habits are subtle everyday things, not dramatic 21-day programs.

In the process, I discovered that I was avoiding activities that ate up my time, such as scrolling, holding protracted phone discussions about unimportant topics, or brooding. I visualized the kind of me who would exercise regularly and eat healthfully. I realized that my days were incredibly customized and would not resemble any other lifestyle videos on the internet. It was okay if something that worked well one day didn't make sense the next.

Last evening, Nolan came in early, just as I was getting ready to try out the new chair cardio moves I had discovered. It was a hectic week for him, and he was in the mood to unwind with beer and munchies. I would normally dump my workout plan to avoid wet-blanketing Nolan's plans. But this time, I continued working out, keeping the conversation going. It took about 15 minutes for Nolan to change and set up the table, and I had done my workout in that time. A small choice determined my actions.

By converting my random smartphone scrolling time to chair yoga time, I managed to devote an unbelievable eight hours every week to working out. Emptying your thoughts is more powerful than cluttering the brain with more stimulus.

On Deciding to Lose Weight

My notes on my food and lifestyle revealed that I was overweight, low on stamina, and undernourished. I had to now define my idea of getting into shape. It was not going to be about weighing less, and I was not going to do anything short-term, drastic, or unsustainable. I was looking for a solution that I saw myself growing gracefully older into, something I would be proud of and would want Hazel to imbibe as she grew up. I wanted to internalize that there was no one isolated magical formula when it came to the amount, style, and variety of food and activity.

I asked myself what I wanted to do in the name of exercise. I didn't get a clear answer.

"Start with something you love doing," Nolan had told me during one of our brainstorming sessions.

I knew I wanted to be by myself and feel safe with the workout. I knew I would do well on my own and did not feel the need to get into a group or community. Yoga, therefore, appealed.

I went to a clinic for basic checkups that Jane said would indicate my yoga readiness. The physiotherapist there green-lighted me for all basic poses but asked me to be cautious about my lower back during advanced poses.

She also mentioned diastasis recti, a condition where the abdominal muscles separate due to all the load they take, especially occurring during pregnancy and childbirth. These muscles could get back to their original structure with some effort. Thanks to my going back to work and sitting most of the time, I put in no effort. This explained the flabby-looking paunch I have still retained.

Chair yoga offered a gentle movement that would engage my abdominal muscles. Diastasis recti is not confined to women alone; men can also develop the condition due to muscle imbalance and incorrect, intense exercises.

"Gee! I seem to have a knowledge deficit in so many areas!" Sitting back and thinking objectively allowed me to see my patterns of faulty attitudes. Going to the doctor and physiotherapist was such a wise place to start, I thought, thanking Jane.

THE ACT OF BEING SEATED

I had yet to understand why the act of sitting, something natural and essential to many jobs, was being so vilified. Anything you read on health viciously attacks the act of sitting, especially at work. Chairs with a backrest have earned notoriety for being the new cigarette.

We sit to work and beat the exhaustion of sitting with more sitting. Reading Daniel Lieberman (2020) helped me summarize the health concerns in these points. Every sitting phase is an opportunity for movement lost, uninterrupted inactivity harmfully elevates sugar and fat levels in the bloodstream, and lastly, hours of sitting might trigger our immune systems to attack our bodies through inflammation, causing slow organ damage. The solution for undoing this harm involves taking frequent breaks when sitting to activate the body systems multiple times, keeping the blood sugar, fat, and inflammation levels low.

This information helped my case for chair yoga and helped me become self-empathetic. I have considered getting a stand-up desk or portable stand tray to work so that I can stand and work whenever I can. I don't want to be in a position where I have to make efforts to begin a pose. I want to be like a ball in motion because a stationary ball is difficult to start rolling.

I AM FINALLY MAKING HEADWAY

Practicing bending forward correctly was the precursor to future poses like the downward dog. I woefully discovered that my spine would not lengthen enough for me to hold many beginner-level poses, which was frustrating.

The forward fold poses were a series that initiated the change for me. Starting with the half-forward fold where the hands take support of the wall or hold the shin bones will get you accustomed to the dynamics. My hamstrings are not yet ready to take the standing forward fold, and this is niggling at my go-getter sensibilities. I wanted to take my time but dreamt of getting this feather in my cap.

I liked the downward dog pose because it instantly energized me, especially when I was anxious. It was a foundational pose; the prone position got the blood flow to my head and calmed me down rather quickly. I kept the chair variation for the office and the floor one for the house to get the best of both. In the initial days, this pose helped me acclimatize to stretches and bends and increase the range of motion of my arms and legs. It particularly helped me with movements of the neck and shoulders. The forward bend opened my chest and allowed for more expansive breathing. Imagine getting a good stretch like a pet dog with no care in the world!

I loved the warrior pose. It got me into combat mode! It essentially symbolized my forceful energy of inner transformation and kindled my ability to convert anger and insecurities into strength and courage. The standing variations are undoubtedly challenging but can be effectively recreated on the chair.

CHAPTER 8

BOLD AND BEAUTIFUL EXPERIMENTS

SCAN FOR AUDIO CHAPTER

10:00 p.m. a plan is in motion

"Hey, Noli, can we look at some diet tweaks for the house? I would love to get your views on our food patterns going forward. Let's try creating a blueprint... come on, come on!"

Nolan was on the chair wearing only a sulky expression and boxers. I had refused to accompany him to the party that weekend. I was secretly enjoying his annoyance, as he went on about how I shouldn't ditch people at the last moment.

We sat down that night to put our thoughts together and had countless conversations about food. We were on the same page with a lot of stuff, but nothing came close to being implemented. It was like a favorite topic for lip service that never translated to action, and of course, we had our justifications for it.

Things, however, became much simpler when we made notes: cut back on sugar, eat more servings of vegetables and fruits per day, avoid carbohydrates later in the day, eat more lean meat and fish, don't feel guilty about occasional indulgences, don't avoid food groups altogether, look for wholesome food over processed ones, stay hydrated, be moderate in practice and opinions.

"Sounds practical," both of us commented at the same time. This time, we also made an action plan to determine what would go permanently off our shopping list, and we decided on meal prep times together like we were planning a holiday. The discussion itself left us satiated, and that deserved a high-five!

Next, I wanted to reevaluate my wardrobe. Functionality influences my shopping patterns now. I would look for designs offering free movement and style. I was surprised at the range in the market!

Ah! That heady feeling of bringing about change.

WHEN NEGATIVE BECOMES POSITIVE

If I ever needed a quick formula to ruffle up Nolan, all I had to do was bring up his pet peeve: dieting. His chatter turns to stifled silence when he senses someone on the "I have been on this diet for the past month" or "Oh I shouldn't be eating carbs now" trip. He abhors discussions that lead to restrictions on intake and thinks they ruin time-tested patterns. He, much to my annoyance, merrily sneers at people who are hung up on their diet plans.

I suspect it has to partly do with his memories of his childhood that were dominated by those of his mom perpetually fretting over what she ate and the mood swings and fights that followed. He persisted with his rather strong view that moderation was key because of the psychological perils he experienced growing up.

We now know that a faulty diet is at the root of many lifestyle issues. What is fascinating is our response patterns. Some of us end up fearing food, feeling the need to take control, and coming up with unsustainable solutions, whilst many of us are curious and want to know more without having to complicate matters.

"I can't get around the idea that there are only certain ways of eating right. Things get messy when we have highly opinionated people flood social media with their limited understanding, influencing our conversations," Nolan would say whenever I confronted him.

"I just find it too simplistic, Mae; I have nothing against anybody having a view, and it is good that people are talking about it. But we forget to look at the biological, emotional, cultural, and psychological aspects of food. People cannot be judged using standard reference points."

"But how does that make things simple?" I was getting impatient.

"I can't help but notice that anxiety is almost always the dominating emotion in the conversation, and is that a good thing? I prefer the body positivity way. What makes anybody think they know how much fat is safe for my body to keep?" Noli was in the mood to lecture today.

"My way of cutting the clutter is this: The food I eat should be harmonious with my emotions, my conditioning, and my health. I would stay away from processed food as much as possible, not get carried away by marketing and packaging, and remain alert to empty calories. We have reached a stage in human history where people are dying of over-nourishment. That is what it is. The only trouble is that it will be a while before people realize this; I rest my case," he concludes with a wink and a grin.

Unapologetic again! I know when it makes sense to give up.

6:00 p.m. all ways lead to wellness

"If the need to fit in is coming from a place of vengeance or fear, then it will lead you nowhere, Maya. The need must arise out of self-love," Jane said.

I needed time to process this. I had to deal with how Bitul's passing comment affected me, especially because I had a lot of emotional gaps. It felt like deadwood continuing to smolder after the fire had been extinguished. My feelings of low self-worth had flared up. I was to now face my inner toxicity and transform it through compassion.

I had to stop berating myself. Expecting my schedules, preferences, and everything I identified with to change fast and giving up at the first obstacle was self-abuse. I began to accept the varying hues of my moods, and it was more therapeutic than I had imagined.

"While practicing yoga, bring variations by including other strength training workouts too," advised Jane.

"Is that not a problem? I thought you would want me to follow one discipline."

"Oh no! Yoga is not the kind of discipline that competes with any other form of training. It will only heighten your self-awareness and make you better at whatever else you are doing. It gives you the mental freedom to be removed from bias. Yoga is about discovering balance, the interplay of strength and tenderness to explore previously undiscovered possibilities of the mind and body."

She continued, "It will only make you efficient at exercising, dancing, or weight lifting—whatever you choose. I don't quite understand the tendency to put down another system to pitch one's own."

I felt assured and invigorated as we walked toward the peaceful pond at the south of Central Park, lined with gleaming schist.

As I removed my mental obstacles, everything fell into place. My clarity of thought allowed me to progress. I had the impression that my surroundings—including my house, workplace, and the people in them—were working in tandem with my goals. I realized that the universe lent itself to a person's intentions, and I grew more and more persuaded by this.

11:30 a.m. an old acquaintance, an old habit

I called up Sam, my trainer. I was afraid he would refuse to get back with me—given the erratic learner I had been. He came over on Saturday evening, ready with a plan for me. I was relieved. When we spoke, he said we would first work on the mindset. He told me about the pattern he had observed in me, and I was thankful he brought it up. It turns out that somewhere in my mind I dread physical workouts because I see them as stressful.

I could not deny it because the memory of school competitions got me emotionally charged. I had seen my friends get humiliated for underperformance. My friend Roni used to skip school on many Thursdays to avoid gym class. I vividly remember the churning in my stomach when the coach walked in with his whistle and notepad to test our skills. Now that I think of it, it's such a pity that for many of us, the definition of physical activity is anything but fun.

I had hold of my first barrier by the collar. I now needed to deploy my resources to manage it. My mental notion of physical activity had to shift to make it deeply personal without external demands and something that gave me solace. To fix this, I had to train to keep my eyes on the prize, remove obstacles from my range of thought, and look at things differently to correct my mental block.

Not having to get out of my chair would be a good start.

OVER THE NEXT FEW WEEKS

I started by congratulating myself on deciding to get my act together amid all the chaos. Using the word "movement" instead of "workout" in my head also helped. Reminding myself to move would then find me looking for opportunities to do so. I would get up to fetch a file instead of requesting Meryl to fetch it and I would help Hazel organize her toys. At times, walking to the store instead of ordering in was my movement. These seemingly insignificant things began to play on my mindset.

I would do small chunks and define my achievements in words. I would end up talking about trivial successes during casual chats in the office and with Nolan.

The next time I tried the hand-to-toe pose, I was better prepared. My nerves did not tense up like before. My brain was sending friendly signals. I used resistance bands to loop around my soles and lift my legs. There was some progress, and I felt encouraged. My body was cautiously lengthening itself and opening up. It was a profound feeling.

I patiently went through the beginner exercises because that would lay the foundation for taking control of my movements. I placed special emphasis on weight loss because it would give me a strong sense of purpose. I had begun modifying my mindset about food and needed a workout plan in place too. Most of all, I needed to love my body the way it was. Yoga would help me overcome this and make me conscious of what I fed my body. So, it would help me get my calorie consumption right, tone my muscles, and teach me patience—I felt like I was on the right track.

I get into the child's pose when I am really tired. Late-night cocktail dinners or long-drawn hearings sometimes leech the energy out of me. The forward fold massages my aching back, while resting my tummy and chest on the cushion as I focus on breathing is inexplicably relaxing. It calms my nerves and helps me sleep very well.

This pose goes well on my work desk too. I pull back my chair a bit, spread my legs a little, check my clothing, and rest my hands and head on the desk to practice. A few seconds of this three to four times a day helps me deal with back pain and hit the refresh button.

My thoughts began to wander. I grew up on a diet of LA Law, Ally McBeal, and stuff that shaped my ideas on what being a lawyer entailed. Those hourglass-figured, immaculately dressed protagonists nowhere reflect my days wherein I barely get to wash my hair regularly. It is what it is.

The lion and the chin lock poses help tone my face. Sticking my tongue out felt strange initially, but I gradually realized how it relaxed my neck muscles. Yoga gave me a much-needed break from screen time—investing a few seconds regularly would surely go a long way.

The downward dog variation while sitting in a chair is a simple calming stretch that gets the blood flowing during long periods of desk work. My capacity to do more repetitions improved, and I felt encouraged.

I also discovered that the high lunge pose was an effective warm-up exercise before I got any further on my chair yoga routine. It worked well on the lower back, gluteus, hips, quadriceps, ankles, and feet. Sciatic nerve stretching helps manage cramps through increased blood flow.

Once you get familiar with the pose on the chair, it is only fair to try it on the yoga mat for a good side stretch. The muscle activity triggered in the lower body will give you a sense of true achievement. As opposed to a low lunge where the knee of the stretched leg touches the ground behind you, this is a more dynamic pose.

The half-fish pose is one hell of a twister. I needed to do enough of the Bharadwaja and Marichi twists to nail this one. The glute muscles get worked up with the crossing, giving you a run for your money. This one especially benefits the spinal cord and is a good workout for stimulating digestion by helping the digestive system secrete juices. The deeply energizing property of the pose makes it a go-to exercise after long hours at the office desk. Do not even think of rushing through this one. You'll feel the blood flow with fresh gusto on twisting.

Mastering Vishnu's couch pose is sure to keep you occupied for days. It took me a good week to even get close to the perfect pose. I like to try this floor pose in the evenings on the play carpet.

Get comfortable with lying on your side with your head supported by your arm. My neck hurt the first time, and I was wobbling away to Hazel's delight. Take time to experience the sensations and feel more balanced.

Once you are okay lying down on both sides, lift one leg straight without bending at the knee. Place your free hand in front of your chest while lifting your leg. Inhale and exhale while lifting and relaxing alternately. Your pelvis will open up better with practice.

Once you have achieved free leg movements, try the final pose where you use your hands to lift your leg by holding the big toe so your leg and hand are vertical to the ground. The day you achieve this will deserve a special celebration.

CHAPTER 9

PICKING UP THREADS

SCAN FOR AUDIO CHAPTER

JUNE: NEW WORK-LIFE BALANCE

Sanders was sheer magic when he spoke, but his body was not cooperating. At 230 lbs, he was struggling with blood pressure and type 2 diabetes. He did not even attempt to hide his weakness for food.

I couldn't help but notice how worn out he appeared. "Sanders, everything's fine? You don't seem like your bright self," I remarked. He took a deep breath and slouched on the chair. Then, he grinned and said, "Life is catching up, Maya." I sensed that he wanted to talk.

"With the high of all this," he waved his hand about, "and everything that comes with it, it has been decades now... but it still motivates me," he said in a low, thoughtful tone. "But when I'm by myself, I feel like I should have done better—personally—not in terms of what one would tend to think. I believe I ought to have been more kind to myself. I was happy with the label of 'workaholic' and didn't give my irregular eating or odd sleeping patterns much thought."

"You know I can't work without smoking, and despite having diabetes, I can't stop drinking Coke. My older one is just 32, and he is already on medication for hypertension. Looking back, I think I should have prioritized right; it's too late."

"Well, that's the way it is!" he said. Regaining his composure and returning to his upbeat self. "Since it's difficult to correct mistakes, I don't want the next generation to make the same ones."

I promised myself it wouldn't.

We left the brand-new conference room of our recently renovated loft-style office. He gave my shoulder an affectionate pat and said, "You will do well, Maya." While I was saying "thank you," Sanders added, "I also like the way young people take care of themselves. What's that girl's name? I admire her... Meryl seems very put together. Such people go a long way."

Sanders had called for a special meeting. The entire team was present at brunch. Whenever he was in the New York office, he would have to bear with Tracy's nagging but didn't mind it in the least or rather enjoyed the digs—they had been colleagues for 30 years now.

Sanders began in his baritone voice, "Guys, amongst other things, we have an agenda. I don't know or care if there is a precedent for this, but we will be here, having weekly brainstorming sessions on putting together a sensible well-being policy for us here at Griffin Law Chambers." That was unexpected, and we got curious.

"I am not looking for standard operating procedures. We know how much they suck. We want a highly customized, need-based system that will be unique to each of us, simply because our circumstances and challenges are different. Let's talk about flexible timings, work-from-home options, negotiable vacation windows, and anything that would give authentic solutions. I am looking for genuine solutions that make sense for the people here."

"Remember, we have no idea how it's going to play out; that's why we need to brainstorm. We will treat people like people, not operating systems."

Oh boy! It was chaos for the next few hours. Sanders-Brown, the true leader he was, had taken the audacious step of wanting to address the issue at the core of everyone's heart. It was challenging because we had to prime ourselves to think differently and approach the project in unconventional ways. It would take some time for the whole idea to sink in. On his way out of the office, with his juniors in tow, he admitted to Tracy, "How I wish I had done things differently from the very beginning."

"It's never too late Sanders," replied Tracy with conviction.

I decided to replace my office chair with an armless design, which gave me a newfound sense of freedom on my path to finding strength, peace of mind, and self-care.

2:30 p.m. a long overdue bonding sesh

I was stretching away when Meryl walked in. That was embarrassing. Do I apologize? You are waiting for a reason to mock yourself... I parroted Jane's words mentally.

"Hey, Meryl! The draft's done?" I passed the whole thing over. I saw her relax at my tone, and we worked away into the afternoon.

"You seem to be taking all this rather well, Meryl." The remark came out of my growing affection for her. The puzzle had finally fallen into place. My initial resentment for her stemmed from the fact that she possessed the very calmness I was longing for. But I was now on the right track, thanks to Jane.

"I remember being a perpetual bundle of nerves when I was an intern. I was convinced that work was all about surviving and dodging one surprise after another."

Meryl's face tightened up, and I sat up not knowing what to expect.

"When I was growing up, it was like that. One trauma followed by another. Perhaps that is why nothing else seems bad."

I pulled my chair close to hers and waited. A lot of memories were clearly stirring up.

"After my father passed away when I was three and my brother was five, my mother had to reinvent herself to run the household. She buried her happy-go-lucky demeanor and made it big as a make-up artist on film sets."

"I grew up seeing her exhausted, and often dejected, at the unforgiving nature of work. Her fears for our well-being led her to make choices that took a toll on her health."

"She would stand countless hours and put up with repetitive strain injuries and her schedules were unpredictable because they depended on a million factors, including the moods of the actors. She wouldn't show her fatigue, but it was not hidden from us. All this before she lost her battle to cancer." Meryl's voice was calm, and her eyes stared into the distance.

"But Mamma was a mature lady, almost spiritual. Having seen the greenroom realities of glamor, she understood the perils of superficial living like nobody else. It got her to bring us up grounded."

"She used to always tell us as kids that no matter what life threw at us, there would be opportunities to discover what we truly wanted from life. She was an optimist despite everything. That spirit gave us our bearings, I guess."

The conversation with Meryl was like taking a cold shower. I promised myself that I would take another look at a lot of things.

MY LITTLE BREAKTHROUGHS

September: Hello to the Sun

It was autumn, and I was more enthusiastically welcoming than I could remember. With great satisfaction, I mused how, in the last few months, I had discovered so much about myself—I almost felt like I had been running like a headless chicken all my life.

Like with beginning anything worthwhile, the initial days were not easy. I felt dull aches and pains in my body and spirit as I treaded unfamiliar grounds. But the discomfort made it a challenge worth overcoming, and eventually, I began tasting triumph.

My morning chair work by the window grew into a sacred retreat, with me sitting serenely on it like a mountain. I got the hang of setting intentions for the day. The deliberateness helped me see where my energies were being diverted and create boundaries—a far cry from my previous default mode of letting the day get to me.

As I did the forward fold pose today, my hip bones willingly lent themselves to the bends and stretches. I could feel the tension release from my neck, shoulders, lower back, and hips as I bent forward to touch the floor with my palms. It also helped me overcome the pain in my tailbone.

This pose activated the glute muscles and hamstrings more gently as compared to standing poses. The blood flow increased toward my head and helped me sleep better. I love doing this pose just after a long car drive.

The pigeon pose was next on my list. My first attempt brought a sharp tension to my hip bones as I crossed my right leg onto my left thigh. I realized I needed to slow down and warm up my legs with gentle movement. I got off the chair and did a few hip-rotation moves. Jane would suggest getting back to the basics if a new pose ever felt difficult. All poses were to begin with warm-ups and breathing exercises and end with relaxation. These were non-negotiable steps.

Last Sunday at the park, Jane introduced me to a sequence called the sun salutation or *surya namaskar*. The morning sun seemed to have stalled to stare at the magic Jane and her yoga students created. One of her students had put on soft meditative music and everyone was on their portable chairs learning the sequence when I landed. It was a series of simple harmonious movements that progressed in a particular pattern, lending itself to modifications on the chair. It was a whole-body exercise that left you feeling accomplished.

The sun salutation is a series of 12 poses, in which some poses are repeated, and provides balance to both sides of the body. It works the nervous system, relaxing the neck, shoulders, and spine, and is an ideal warm-up sequence. The rhythmic flow and stretch lubricate your joints. It expands the chest muscles and improves respiration. It also helps balance emotions by bringing in a sense of harmony with nature. I was asked to be slow and deliberate with my movements to soak in every progression.

The cobra pose helps open up the middle and upper back along with your chest muscles. I am susceptible to spondylitis, so I am slow with my movements. Bending backward invariably invites discomfort, so I take my time to feel the effects of the movements. Jane believes it helps the thyroid glands. The pose also helps me overcome the bloated feeling in my stomach. It is my go-to pose when feeling lethargic a few hours after a heavy meal.

The dolphin pose is a floor-based yoga pose that helps tone your biceps and shoulders and open up your chest muscles. I like doing this pose at home in the mornings on my yoga mat and in the evenings on the carpet while spending time with my daughter. Also known as the half-feathered peacock pose, this is one of those all-around poses that help you feel refreshed. Since the body weight shifts to the arms and upper body, it adds vitality by inducing reverse blood flow, and I look forward to doing this regularly because I like the feeling of achievement it gives me each time.

I appreciate the uniqueness of each new pose I learn and realize that the process and outcome are nothing like what you see in a picture of the poses. You begin to feel the nuances of the experiences each time you do the poses. They have a life and message of their own that cannot be shared through words or demonstrations.

4:00 p.m. some me-time

This evening, I craved a good head massage and a yogurt hair pack to pamper myself. I left the pack on for 40 minutes and looked for a relaxing pose. The half-frog pose is a good back-bending floor pose that strengthens your hips, quadriceps, ankles, chest, and shoulders and improves overall flexibility.

The "half" in any pose suggests an asymmetric pose. Your side abdominal muscles, hamstrings, glutes, and pelvis are intensely engaged for a full-body workout. You can feel the weight of your body on your abdomen and hips, which helps you get a better sense of balance. The abdominal organs and the adrenal glands are stimulated due to the prone position.

I love doing this after I have been sedentary either at work or at a party to relax my neck and spine. Changing into comfortable pajamas, letting your hair down, and lying on the carpet for some stretches is the most relaxing idea after a long day.

The pyramid pose is a deep forward fold pose done with or without a chair as an aid. It is great for stretching your spine and hamstrings. Its non-intrusive form allows you to do it in the most restrictive of environments and has helped me overcome the most stressful situations in the office. I just let my head fall and connect to my body and mind deeply.

I highly recommend a few warm-ups before doing the pyramid pose because it demands some intense back and hamstring stretching. Taking the first step back to form a triangle gave me a jolt on my first attempt. I felt myself wobbling and unable to maintain my balance. I was not in complete harmony with my body. I practiced by holding onto the backrest of the chair and gradually proceeded to do it independently. My abdominal muscles felt toned and contracted after every practice.

I went on to try the *surya namaskar* since it was a full-body pose. It was supposed to provide enthusiasm and energy to face the day ahead, making you conscious of your innate strength. It would help channel my strengths and relax my nerves.

Stretching my arms and legs, twisting my waist in particular, and holding the position turned out to be tough for me. I was a bit unsettled by this failure. However, I remembered Jane's instructions to direct my full attention to the pain area to avoid overdoing the stretches. I had to know when to stop and learn to differentiate between a positive and harmful push.

So much work was yet to be done. I had lost the flexibility and stamina of my early years. It was a discouraging feeling. A simple pose stumped me, and I knew I needed to get my act together.

For starters, I decided to practice the correct sitting position to get my spine erect. I needed a healthy mix: cardiovascular workouts to keep my lungs and heart strong; strength training to build muscle and strengthen joints; and stretching to develop muscle flexibility. I made a mental note. Strategies had to be drawn. The case was challenging!

CHAPTER 10

LOSING IT WITH LOVE

SCAN FOR AUDIO CHAPTER

1:30 p.m. I think I found a new role model

I began to keep track of the sheer amount of time I spent on body image thoughts. All conversations would invariably veer toward weight issues. At the office, at college reunions, at family get-togethers, at the dinner table, over coffee... it was endless. Comments like, "Hey, have you lost weight?" or seeing them biting their tongue but betraying with looks that they think you have put on weight were commonplace.

We know that fad diets don't work but can't resist attempting the latest buzz in the market, hoping it will work this time. We also admit to needing to eat wholesome food but do the opposite, with justifications of course. We consume fitness videos day in and day out but don't spend even a quarter of the time putting what we see into practice.

What struck me was the inertia of it all. It was like an unspoken agreement—a collective consciousness toward inaction—or more of a reconciliation about body weight issues. "I am not happy with my state of affairs—neither are you and nor is anybody; let's go back to work."

We all had the same message posted on our brows. We never talked ourselves into acting; we just wanted to hear why we were the way we were. We resisted any solution. Anybody who offered solutions would be shut down as we did with Tracy in the office. I was quick to dismiss her; why didn't I simply understand that she made certain choices when she was my age and is reaping the benefits at 50?

Tracy said, "I started bringing the lunch everyone teases me about 25 years ago. I learned as a young mother that cooking was a great way to switch off. I got into a trance twice a day, which offered the mental fuel that kept me sane. I cannot imagine forgoing the everyday cleaning, chopping, and mixing process."

"You make it sound so exotic, Tracy. You describe cooking as one would describe holidaying. I am tempted to copy you," I said to her.

But does that mean bringing a lunch box to work is the only solution? I knew it would take me time to enjoy cooking as she does.

"Bringing a lunch box to work is not the only solution though," she continued as if she read my mind. "You can choose to do that or choose where you eat, but you will have to look for healthy options, and that takes some effort.

"It would mean discovering a smaller food joint and passing over the closest fast-food restaurant, which could perhaps be more expensive," I added.

"Absolutely!" said Tracy. "I was bullied for being overweight as a kid. I fell into a pattern of self-blame, punishing myself for things that were not in my control. I would refuse to let myself be happy, believing I could only do so after I had achieved my ideal body image. I was left miserable and friendless."

"That all changed when I had my girls." She smiled slightly and continued. "I didn't want them to be like me, not knowing how to be kind to themselves. I wanted to be a healthy role model. So, I got help, unlearned my thought patterns, and made my choices. It is amusing how words can sometimes change your life. My therapist's answer to my question about weight loss was, 'The path to weight loss is through health gain'. This notion unknotted several wires in my brain," her smile brightened, and I could feel the sense of relief those words still brought her.

I regretted not trying to know her better all these years.

"I wonder why I resisted my intentions of getting health tips from you, Tracy. It's a gross underutilization of resources, I must say." My newfound excitement was evident.

"Do you find yourself resistant to pick up a book from that shelf?" asked Tracy with a glint in her eyes.

I chuckled. "Of course not! I've not yet succumbed to total inertia."

"Then perhaps you could fetch the Law of Torts for me."

"You are so wicked!" I protested and jumped up to fetch the book.

ON DESIGNING MY DAYS

I admire the conviction youngsters display in their YouTube channels and Instagram posts. I need to find a way to make it work for me in a way that lasts a lifetime. Social media only shows what is chosen to be shown.

If I were to divide things into two baskets—work and life, then exercise and diet would go into my work basket because they need deliberate planning and decision-making and are areas where I can't wait for inspiration to strike.

People with great fitness routines like Tracy maintain them by working toward daily goals with every choice made. I would be naive to think she did it because she had the luxury of doing so. Scores of people with more luxury wouldn't do what she does. I want self-care to be a ritual and a culture I can claim as my own.

I was not ignorant and knew the problem needed to be reevaluated. Finally, the lawyer in me was at work, sifting the truth from truthiness!

Many things we read and hear have the quality of truthiness because we tend to develop beliefs or perceptions without regard for evidence, logic, intellectual examination, or facts, or they could be largely ignorant assertions of deliberate propaganda intended to sway opinions like the media does through advertisements.

I needed to work on my beliefs and attitudes toward situations and people. I needed to respond appropriately to the transient. I didn't want to compromise work. I wanted to spend every other moment at home with Hazel during her formative years. I needed to be relaxed and not perpetually tick off my to-do lists.

ON HOW EXERCISE AFFECTS THE BRAIN

Targeted research by Suzuki (2017) revealed how mood enhancements brought on by each bout of exercise aided the brain over time in maintaining attention and focus for longer than usual periods and resulted in enhanced memory and energy.

Through this particular study, the cumulative effects of exercise on brain function have come into focus, thus fundamentally altering how we think about exercise. Moving your body has a strong transformational effect on the brain. Raising levels of neurotransmitters including dopamine, serotonin, and noradrenaline has an instant impact. Focus is improved after just one workout, and the effects last for at least two hours.

Additionally, it speeds up your response time. The brain's structure, physiology, and function change throughout time due to the creation of new brain cells, which enhances memory and attention. The prefrontal cortex and hippocampus are protected against neurodegenerative diseases associated with aging, which is the most significant benefit.

7:30 p.m. same living room, new me

Hazel was watching me suspiciously and getting rather amused at my twists and turns. She will get used to it in the coming days. It was much better than seeing me lying on the couch or scrolling mindlessly.

As I sat on the carpet with Hazel, I noticed I couldn't squat. The hips and calf muscles were stiff and hurt badly, and I lost balance in a matter of minutes. Wow! A lot needs to be done! I hope my girl will grow up with a strong body and not compromise on her physical abilities. As she played, I got onto a chair and decided to do a few more poses.

NOT FORGETTING TO LOVE ONESELF

I never thought of office lunch planning, especially the menu, as something that should concern me Maria always ordered the food. The takeaway joints were tried and tested, and the menu comprised typical fan favorites that everybody would surely eat. This time, however, I found myself checking with her, "Fancy ordering in from that new joint, Maria? They claim to be serving a 'healthy, wholesome' menu."

When the food came, everybody noticed the change and wondered if Tracy had a hand in this! The new menu won everybody's hearts, and it was an unexpected triumph for me. Even Sanders said he didn't miss the Coke this time.

I needed to get myself to a place where I would eat something because I wanted to, not because I had a compulsive habit that I needed to get out of.

5:00 p.m. learning something new about food

"You will not believe me. I love food. I do not count calories and am indulgent when I get my favorite dishes. Food has emotional aspects attached to it. We have an increased appetite when in good company or on a happy occasion. I will reach for something French when I am on an emotional low," said Jane.

"Do you feel emotionally low after all these years of yoga?" I asked.

"Yes, of course. Yoga doesn't numb you. In fact, it makes you acutely aware of yourself and equips you to handle things effectively. There is a difference," she replied.

"Don't complain that I am preaching," Jane elaborated. "We are more likely to be harsh with ourselves and don't feel the need to be self-compassionate despite knowing how important it is. The words and tone we use when talking to ourselves are very different from what we use when talking to others."

There are, in theory, many solutions; keep your mind open to them. We figure things out and evolve at different levels—personally and collectively. We feed off each other's experiences, and that is beautiful. Chair yoga is the easiest to integrate into your reality. Most of us are already by or on a chair several times a day.

My first experience with sitting still was unsuccessful. But I realized that I found it difficult to sit still without any apparent purpose. That is important information, and I need to figure out how to move forward from here.

You may not perceive the correlation between chair yoga and weight loss right now. It's fine to be skeptical. In sitting still with ourselves and focusing on our breath, we learn to heighten the awareness of our body and mind.

We brush aside or stifle a lot of sensations, especially when we are occupied with important things. We lose our ability to sense signals that our bodies and minds send us constantly. We don't know when our stomachs signal that they are full or our spinal cords signal that a pose is hurting. We stifle happiness, joy, fear, and grief, all for being "normal, functional" people.

To address weight issues, we need to first understand their causes. For that, we need to be physically, emotionally, psychologically, and socially aware. Focusing on your breath without being distracted or disturbed is the first step. Sit with your experiences, don't deny them. This will take time, and you must be willing to give it that time.

We associate action with efficiency and results and reject anything slow and sustainable, dismissing them as boring and ineffective. We learn this from everyone and everything around us. Parenting, education, and societal expectations all sing the same tune, except that it appears to be working while destabilizing us at a deeper level.

Does that mean we go about rejecting and rebelling? Yes—not in a dramatic sense but in extremely subtle ways.

"Choosing to eat natural, wholesome food over processed ones, meal after meal, is an example of a huge silent rebellion," Jane grinned. "You will pay the price, mind you.

Food may not be available because you didn't have time to cook, it may not be appealing, it may be expensive or cumbersome to source or not storable, and it may feel funny to consume in social gatherings. But once your objective is clear and awareness present, your mind will begin to provide creative solutions without drawing eyeballs or facing embarrassment. We dread feeling out of place and being noticed for unusual behavior—it's understandable.

Baked potatoes stand no chance against pineapple tarts under normal circumstances. You may feel tired or your sugar levels may be low, but that's when your willpower needs to shine. With severe conflict in your mind and no time, you can't be caught staring at the food or contemplating for too long without you or people wondering what you are up to. Your emotions, body, and mind oppose your intellect. So, we have the rider and the hungry elephant. It's a no-brainer situation here. If you pass the tart and pick the potatoes, you will have stressed yourself, and that is going to burst out somewhere else sometime. Willpower is a depleting resource. It's just too taxing to sustain. It is only a matter of time!

If you had heightened awareness, you would not have let your sugar levels deplete in the first place. Matching your food intake with your work would help you avoid becoming the hungry elephant. Even if you were hungry, you would have reached out for the tart out of choice and been happy about the choice, not feeling guilty. You would then reset the cost with logical actions and be better prepared to face such a situation the next time it happens.

Heightened awareness allows us to naturally reject excess food because the body's signals will be activated. This makes weight loss a natural consequence. The notion that you need to beat yourself up with tough workouts and food deprivation will simply not stick.

You can blame the fitness industry for making you believe that you need to purchase workout and diet programs. These are intrinsic capabilities we no longer know how to harness. We have reached a stage where we refuse to believe that things can be simple. I do not go shopping when I have not eaten for a long time because I would buy something tempting for sure or waste my quota of willpower.

Misconceptions continue floating around. Not to blame people across the board, but yes, we cannot afford to be naive enough to believe everything.

Where in the work–life balance we all love talking about would you place exercises? The life side, of course.

But exercise is work. The body is good to go without exercise. Physical activity is entirely voluntary and a choice just like your career. Therefore, it needs to be on the work side and will require the same amount of effort to sustain. Exercise is not natural for the body, so you will never feel intrinsically motivated to do it. It has to be thrust into your day. That's the fundamental understanding we need to internalize, and our approach changes when we do so. As far as the body is concerned, exercise is an unnecessary exertion.

WHAT I LEARNED ABOUT BODY FAT

I perceived body fat to be such a monster that I completely forgot that they are essentially tissues that store energy and protect the body. My approach to managing fat would depend on what I understood about it. I aimed to increase my metabolism and avoid excess storage to help shrink cell size. I had to find a way to burn the fat that was getting stored, and working my muscles was the answer to that.

Otherwise, I would be looking to shorten the process through harmful means. If I took random pills that promised fat loss, I needed to know what they did biologically; my obsession with the bathroom scales also lessened when I learned about the fat-to-muscle ratio.

If I ate less to lose weight, I would lose fat and lean mass, and losing lean mass is not healthy. But if I maintained my protein intake and burned fat by building muscle through resistance training, I would reduce only fat and retain muscle tissue. When I get to keep my muscle tissue, I retain the possibility of burning fat. Why? Because only muscles have the capability of burning fat.

ON WHY HIGH-INTENSITY INTERVAL TRAINING (HIIT) WORKS WELL AND THE SCIENCE BEHIND IT

Subjecting our bodies to high-intensity workouts at regular intervals makes us strong, fit, fast, and healthy. HIIT is essentially intense cardiovascular spurts that demand a lot from our bodies. It makes you sore post-workout but develops stronger, thicker muscle by changing its fiber composition. It also enables your muscles to transport glucose from the bloodstream and produce more energy.

HIIT results in lower blood pressure and helps ward off lifestyle issues. It also increases your heart's ability to pump blood efficiently by improving the elasticity of its chambers and arteries. HIIT is highly recommended for athletes and average people.

MY INTRODUCTION TO HIIT

Chair-cardio workouts are high-movement, high-energy workouts when compared to the slow and deliberate yoga poses I regularly do. I love combining both for variety and fun. The movements listed here are my favorites and can be done in combinations for five-minute high-intensity sessions at least a couple of times a day.

Cardiovascular HIIT workouts made me break into a sweat and tested my stamina. After overcoming the initial discomfort, I looked forward to doing them often. The first trials were uncomfortable, no doubt, but I began getting better as I worked on my mindset to own the process. I would allow myself to feel like Hazel: Happy without a reason.

As with chair yoga poses, we had to warm up the pelvic area gradually with upper and lower body movements before going into movements that called for twisting, bending, and extending. Use chair cardio to boost your metabolism and trigger calorie burning without moving out of your workstation.

The important thing is to avoid progressing to high-movement exercises if you've been sitting stiffly for a long time. It's a good idea to stand up and do a bit of walking around once in a while. This will help prevent sprains and injury.

I would get carried away looking at exercise videos. All the moves looked super simple to watch but turned out to be a different story when I attempted to recreate them with my body. Expectations did not match reality, and I had to avoid getting impatient.

The inclusion of HIIT 'how-to' instructions and illustrations are outside the scope of this book however, they are provided in the free bonus booklet (page 257).

CHAPTER 11

LOOKING FOR THE PERFECT RECIPE

SCAN FOR AUDIO CHAPTER

October: Monday, 2:00 p.m. we're different yet same

Selena admitted, "There was no way I could not have swiped my card. I mean she was THE angel who I had finally stumbled upon because of good karma. She knew my deepest pain points, how my attempts at exercise had not worked, that I had no time, and that I was frustrated with years of failure. She spoke at length about how her research and sweat and blood had paid off in developing just the right program for ME. I paid up, got the resources, read, and started my sure-to-succeed journey." She was pouring her heart out as she frantically picked up papers and stuffed them inside the folder.

"And then what happened?" I asked, trying to suppress my grin, knowing it was a triggering question. Selena, my colleague, and a buddy, gave me her spiteful look, hating me for having asked, and very expectedly, broke down. "Well, maybe I am a born failure. Nothing seems to work for me." She pushed off her chair to pick up the file she had dropped.

"Yoga? Chair...but I said weight loss, darling!' she shot back at my suggestion.

"There is no one coming to rescue you, babe. You need to take the onus. How long are you going to wait for magic? Stop believing that somebody else has a secret you need to pay to access. Every time you find yourself hating the process of getting in shape, know that it is unhealthy in any case," I persisted.

"Selena, dear, I do not mean disrespect to that program. They all have relevant information. But not everything wonderful in and of itself is necessarily applicable to your circumstances, and it takes more to make something work. Will purchasing programs, paraphernalia, and memberships benefit you?"

"Having a fitness trainer works for me because it operates on a very human level. The lively talks and connections bring a lot of significance, which help me focus and sustain. But a few years ago, when my challenges looked different, I could not have said this. I had to figure out what workouts I could do and when because of the baby," I tried explaining to her. Knowing my bestie, all I can say is she wouldn't listen.

I could read Selena like the back of my hand. We seemed to have absolutely nothing in common nor could we agree on anything. She lived on the edge, thanks to her refusal to slow down, her belief that life is to be lived on impulses, and her extreme highs and lows. Her secret life had too many secrets to salt away. I couldn't decide what exasperated me more: her many trips to Las Vegas, the weekend high-end parties she'd come back sloshed from, or her numerous risky affairs. We perhaps saw each other as our alter-egos, each filling in for the other's quirk.

There were periods when she looked fabulously fit. She would strut around in designer wear looking on top of the world. However, I would sense that her emotions and state of mind did not match her external fitness.

"Have you been eating less? Have you been exerting yourself to reach your weight loss goal, Selena? Stop ruining your health in the name of fitness, you nut," I would be ruthless with her as she went about pretending everything was fine. She would glare at me only to soon admit I was correct.

"Whatever you said just feels so wrong. You don't want to ever encourage me. You are the bane of my life, you devil!" she yelled.

"Thanks for the compliment—much appreciated. Can we please show up at the trial on time? The judge is not going to wait for you," I said as I dragged her toward the car.

I am certainly suspicious of diet programs that make you dependent on products. I do not like the feeling in my gut when I am told I have been doing things wrong and now need to course-correct them before disaster strikes. The marketing just does not align with common sense. I am very interested in knowing their long-term effects and sustainability and would call any regimen a success only if it helped me feel good over decades and not just a few days. The confusion created around food has so many of us paralyzed.

During break hours, we loved gossiping about diet and fitness across the board. The sheer amount of energy spent on the volley of opinions, contradictions, and advice was extremely entertaining every single time. Intense debates on what is the ideal workout, which is the best exercise wear, what is the most sensible diet, which are the best gyms in town, what are good results, what is the ideal time frame, what paraphernalia you need, and more... the list is endless. I suspect we show more enthusiasm and get a high from talking about fitness to the point of obsession than actually practicing it.

The conversations had to be nudged toward discussing actionable plans. I would encourage Tracy to share tips on interesting recipes, and we would take notes. This would lead Selena to share her experience with successfully carving time out for morning walks. I would pitch in with how I managed to find three hours of no-gadget time every evening. We soon formed a mutually trusting group where we could admit to our failures and course-correct misconceptions.

THE ESSENTIAL INGREDIENTS OF A FITNESS PLAN

While I agonized over my body image, I failed to realize that apart from me, nobody else was judging me for the way I looked. People recognized me for my capabilities, but I was only seeing my many faults—nothing unnatural there, just my approach making change inefficient. I would give space, kindness, and empathy to others but not to myself; I had a toxic relationship with myself. I had to learn to set realistic and simple goals for myself and, more importantly, allow others to help me.

There was me and there was this cliched image of a healthy person that I carried in my head. If I were to be the image in my head, I would be waking up at 4 a.m., working out rigorously, following a vegan diet, being seen at marathons, and losing pounds at will, all while not compromising on being a full-time attorney and mother.

I couldn't seem to conjure the idea of a real person who was well rested, had healthy eating and exercising habits, and could manage the ups and downs with some magnanimity. This everything-or-nothing philosophy affected my emotional health, but I didn't know how to approach things another way. I wanted to jog every day, fix up healthier meals, and avoid sitting so much... all these wants were eating me up. I was perpetually frustrated, had occasional panic attacks at not being able to live up to my expectations, and thought nothing about sounding cynical.

5:30 p.m. a note on empathy

"If this state of mind is your starting point to fitness, you've probably hit the wrong road," said Jane. "Wellness is the precursor to fitness, and this includes a feeling of serenity in multiple areas of life. We put too much energy into physical health," she continued.

I unfairly judged myself based on my physical appearance and got away with it because I found support in the popular rhetoric. As writer Jeanette Winterson observed, "We live in a society that peddles solutions, whether it is solutions to those extra pounds you are carrying, or to your thinning hair, or your loss of appetite, loss of love. We are always looking for solutions, but actually what we are engaged in is a process throughout life during which you never get it right. You have to keep being open, you have to keep moving forward. You have to keep finding out who you are and how you are changing, and only that makes life tolerable." (A Quote by Jeanette Winterson, n.d.).

Kara Wutzke (2021) showed me why empathy needs to be deployed to materialize my weight loss and fitness dreams. I needed to be mentally prepared for setbacks and deal with them instead of beating myself up.

I needed to remind myself perpetually that Nolan, Jane, Sam, Hazel, and my friends were my constant supporters. I had to get the ingredients right if I wanted a good dish!

THE CHICKEN OR EGG STORY: WEIGHT OR METABOLISM?

I was more convinced by the day that my metabolism was worsening due to aging, which was leading to weight gain. It was time to boost my metabolism and get it to behave.

Metabolism is the process of converting all the food we eat and drink into energy. So, the assumption that when food does not get converted to energy due to a weakened metabolism it gets stored as body fat is an appealing argument. Let us question that assumption for a moment and see what comes out of it.

The calories in the food need oxygen to be converted into energy. The body needs a lot of energy just to maintain itself, even in a seemingly inactive state like sitting or sleeping. If there is excess fat in the body, it comes in the way of calorie burning. Body fat accumulation is a direct result of food intake.

Weight gain may result from hyperthyroidism, genetics, lifestyle, and conditions like Cushing syndrome that mirror excess cortisol presence. Metabolism is a complex robust mechanism that does not rely on our decision-making capabilities. In other words, you cannot hasten or slow down your metabolism enough to manage your weight.

As such, life has given us clear enough messages that food intake may be all we can control. It is asking us to keep away from trying to tweak natural bodily functions. The next time you see claims of products or processes that help "boost your metabolism," know that there is no science to back it, and it would only "boost" their market with the bonus of harmful side effects to your body.

Things in my control are ensuring that my food intake does not exceed my calorie expenditure and facilitating excess calorie burning by getting good sleep and performing regular aerobic activities and strength training.

Our bodies are intelligent and will reset their functions to adapt to our intake. So, if I think I can lose weight by consuming fewer calories, my body will readjust its functions to utilize fewer calories. This will result in low energy, more fat storage, increased hair loss (because it isn't critical for survival), and more such untoward changes.

With a basic understanding of science, I could safely conclude that excess weight comes in the way of optimum metabolism and not the other way around. There goes my hope that I am in complete control. All my secret plans of blaming my metabolism for not cooperating with my weight loss plan had to be shelved.

ON THE MISTAKES I HAVE BEEN MAKING WHEN EXERCISING

A few days into my morning routine, I found sitting on the chair for too long uncomfortable. It got tiring and demotivating, and I was fed up with trying. On Sam's direction, I started eating fruit or some nuts before I began the session to allow my body to invest more in the things I do to burn more calories. It helped a little.

He also asked me to avoid doing the same poses continuously, as the neuromuscular pathways get exhausted with monotonous workouts and insufficient opportunities for recovery.

"Your body may reach a peak with a particular exercise, and it won't need to put in the same effort as before to perform it. Regular variations are, therefore, crucial. A lot of my trainees start to resist change, and that's when I know they are entering a demotivation zone," said Sam.

I was over-enthusiastic on some days and overwhelmed on others. Time and again, I slipped into my hard-wired, everything-or-nothing mindset. Keeping it simple and consistent was my challenge.

Warming up with simple poses readies my muscles, heart, and blood pressure for the movements that were to follow. Just like our minds need rest, taking at least a day's break allows our bodies to respond effectively to workouts through optimum recovery.

Errors in judgment and mistakes are as real as successes. Overlooking or denying this has been throwing me off track. I would push myself on a given day and pay the price over the next few days. I had to train myself to listen to my body. Soreness was a sign that the exercise was working, but the pain was another thing.

During the initial days, I would sometimes skip warm-ups or the foundational poses and jump to a newfound pose. The result would be exacerbated joint pain or a muscle pull that would hinder me from doing any poses for a week. I concluded that the best approach, especially to avoid developing incorrect obstructive strategies, was to follow Jane and Sam's advice.

I could do well reading good books on the human body and mind, learning to sift information, and being a learner. I would have to resist the temptation to come to fixed conclusions and be aware of the need to constantly evolve.

CHAPTER 12

GAIN WITHOUT PAIN–I'M LOVING IT!

SCAN FOR AUDIO CHAPTER

I looked at the email again—college reunion. Wait a minute; has it already been a year? I can't believe I have been on my me-project for this long. "Awesome, man! I need to take stock," I blurted out, making a quick note.

In the past year, I began to see the excitement of the process rather than a wish to reach a future ideal state. Things had changed: I refused to be led by fear and used my strengths instead. I deployed my spirit of inquiry to seek facts instead of perceptions. Building my knowledge of the basics of nutrition and exercise is helping me make sensible decisions.

What else? I have stopped being afraid—of food and my body. Since I don't feel powerless around them anymore, I have a sense of control. I have gone through the psychological perils of random diets and have no desire for an encore. I only lost my self-worth in the process, not fat.

Moreover, for the first time, I have begun to look at food as a source of joy, abundance, and nourishment rather than a necessary evil. The one decision I had to make was to go from processed food to whole food. My relationship with my body is finally optimistic, forgiving, and harmonious.

Nolan, Hazel, and I have started going for daily strolls in the evening. We never did that before, and I can't find enough words to describe the good it has done for us. In our half-hour stroll, we soak in the bliss of being together and talk about everything under the sun.

The most challenging of all has been carving out me-time. I had to peel off layers of deep-seated beliefs—it was more complex than I had suspected—and close the gap between knowing and doing—I now know this has to be done with kindness and unconditional support for myself. I am training for that. When I cook, it is for the joy of life. My workout is self-indulgence time, and I do it for the pleasure and peace it gives me. I have learned to marvel at the unpredictability of moments now that I don't go about wanting to control everything about myself.

I had a brief waiting at my desk on Monday morning. Sanders wanted me to consider taking it up because it was from one of our long-standing clients. I studied the file and felt a surge of excitement. I reached out to reply to his mail and started typing out my response, "I would love to jump in." However, I paused mid-sentence and realized my mind was going in a different direction. I contemplated the trade-offs on my calendar and listened.

I composed a polite response, expressing my inability to take up the assignment and my offer to help with delegation. I received a thumbs-up from Sanders in less than an hour. I have perhaps not felt so empowered in a long time. I keep my daily goals simple and find myself achieving more.

Of late, I find myself saying "no" to a lot of stuff I would previously jump at. When I achieve what I commit to, I take my time to soak in the upliftment it brings. I like this feeling of being happy with small successes and not perpetually overwhelmed by all my tasks.

A random thought came to me this morning and wouldn't leave until I paid it attention. It went like this: I assumed that I was not choosing to live a super busy life. But my choice to work hard to prove my worth was a choice I made due to the expectations I set for myself. I now live with that choice and bear its consequences. However, the realization that I can make a different choice and include self-care in it seeped in along with an appreciation that such a change would set me up for positive consequences by default. I liked this idea and couldn't wait to work on it.

I have learned that I pay the price when my commitments to others are fulfilled at the cost of my happiness. It affects my relationships. I have experienced the consequent loss of harmony and do not want to stay in that loop anymore.

9:00 a.m. following in mum's footsteps

I like to begin my days with a plan, and of course, they go haywire. If anything has changed, it's my response. Tracking how I react and thinking about my patterns has helped, giving me ideas on adopting approaches that can help me do what needs to be done.

I begin my day by cleaning, not the house but my thoughts. I have recently developed this pleasurably addictive habit of decluttering. It began with my wardrobe and spilled over to my emails and the work desk. This ritual is rewiring my functioning.

My childhood recollections of laughing uncontrollably while watching Full House include my mom humming in the kitchen in the background. She once used the term "progressive cleaning" to describe her way of keeping the kitchen spotless at all times, and it caught on. She had figured out that I was in my most receptive mood when I laughed and took the opportunity to sneak in her motherly advice. After 30 years, I finally realized that I could employ progressive cleaning to go about my daily life too.

MY INITIATION TO THE SQUEAKY NEW WORLD OF RESISTANCE BANDS

Sam walked in with something fancy yesterday. He brought out these rolls of latex in different sizes from his backpack.

"Here, these are the new-gen dumbbells," he said, handing them over to me.

"You're kidding, right, or are dumbbells into yoga nowadays?"

"Do I laugh at the lame joke?" he asked, amused.

"Seriously, we are going to use them to get your muscles well-toned and strong," Sam added when I continued to stare at him like this was a prank. "You wouldn't come to the gym, and you can compromise on building muscle mass. These resistance bands are going to do a similar job as weights in strength training. No more excuses about a lack of time and bulky equipment," said Sam, handing me a thin loop, which he said was a beginner-level half-inch band.

"You mean there are levels in bands too?" I was keen to know how these wiggly things were going to stand up to the solid dumbbells and humongous machines. I can smell a David and Goliath story somewhere in here!

"They offer low, medium, and high tension to the muscles. Why don't you have a go at this one? I want you to see its magic." Sam reminded me of my tricks at getting Hazel to do some number games—enticing someone to do something they had no clue about!

Following Sam's demonstration and warm-ups, I did a chest pull-apart, feeling the tension in my upper arms and chest initially, and as I pulled further, my upper back muscles came alive. Next were the lateral pulls for the latissimus dorsi muscles found in the sides of the back. I could do them either seated or standing. The band bicep curls had me stepping on the band and pulling it up like the good old curl with weights. My muscles were working the same way that they would when lifting weights.

Sam told me it would build endurance in all my muscle fibers. "It does remind me of weights in the gym... I'm sold."

In the process, I discovered something fascinating about bands. They offer a different kind of resistance than dumbbells or machines, making them more advantageous.

When I used a dumbbell to perform a bicep curl, the action became less difficult as it neared its conclusion because the biceps were no longer being worked as much at this point. This occurred because the length of the lever shortened toward the finish, and the resistance was no longer provided due to gravity's downward pull as the weight sat on your biceps.

In contrast, because resistance increased as you pulled the band, it did not get any easier at any point; you have to work harder to keep the squeeze. This is referred to as "accommodating resistance," and it allows you to advance limitlessly in your workout. The further you pull, the more these latex bands provide resistance. I have to admit that's a fantastic deal.

I was pretty pleased with this discovery and knew resistance training would be worthwhile. For my age, I needed a realistic plan to maintain bone strength and muscle health. More muscle mass meant burning more calories and, hence, would do my metabolism a lot of good.

Bands have a good range of workouts for the upper and lower body. A simple squat provided with a dose of resistance much to my delight. I liked the sidestep squats for their effectiveness in simple movement. My glutes and hips got an intense supported stretch. Eventually, I got familiar with the bands and found them effectively mimicking a lot of equipment I had used at the gym.

8:30 p.m. can't resist these bands

"Let me tell you this. I have come to love resistance bands. I delightfully discovered that I could change the resistance of one band to many levels by widening my feet or pulling at it in different positions with my hands to adjust the stretch. Isn't that efficient? I'll show it to you," I gushed to Nolan at the dinner table as we gossiped about the day.

7:30 a.m. a little more about bands

"How come you don't ask me about numbers, Maya? I am used to answering questions on stats like "how many pounds would that be,""how many reps should I be doing now… I did so many last week,""or do you think I am progressing?" asked Sam.

"I guess it is about what you feel. I like to enjoy the process and look at the big picture… accept my present level as it is and aim for the next possible level." I surprised myself with my answer and realized that my attitude was changing for the good.

"Can I move on to thicker bands for this, Sam?"

"I think it will help you to do this in proper form with a lower resistance than struggling without a smooth pose at the next level, Maya," came his prompt reply. In time, I learned to choose technique over tension—quality over quantity.

"My clients are less intimidated by the bands. Most of them give up on weights rather quickly," he rued.

A useful piece of trivia I love to share with my friends is about how using gloves has helped sustain my workouts without any hassle. I would give up midway since the latex would generate friction on my palms, but with gloves, there is no such thing to stop me. I love to see the improvisations Sam comes up with every single time.

Every time I was careless about removing the band after an activity, my hand would be pulled down as the band would snap back. I am now cautious and go about releasing the band with controlled movements. I also take intervals of a day or two for muscle recovery as with weight training. I wouldn't risk forgetting to modify the intensity to suit my body. Every time I practice a new move, I have to be mindful of how my body is taking it; getting carried away is always a costly affair.

The inclusion of resistance band exercise 'how-to' instructions and illustrations are outside the scope of this book, however, I've listed my go-to resistance band exercises in the free bonus download (page 257).

WHY HAVING STRENGTH BECOMES MORE IMPORTANT AS WE GROW OLDER

I met my extended family once in a blue moon when there was perhaps a wedding. I do, however, have memories of staying over at my grandparents' place in Lyons when I was off from school and bored at home. Mamma would drop me over at Granny's, and I would spend my days lazing around, enjoying the pampering, and taking long walks with Grandpa over the winding roads every evening.

Looking back now, I realize our definitions of self-care are constructed using what we imbibe from our immediate environment. My retired parents take long walks every evening and that keeps them happy. Some aunts here or another uncle there are into sports; they are exceptions to the rule.

The point is that walking has culturally become the definition of exercise. Generally, there is no other exertion of the body because there is no such requirement to live a functional life. I have not seen real people around me adopt strength training and other forms of working out as a ritual. This explains my natural skepticism and reluctance to adopt anything else into my own life. If this has to change for the next generation, we need to set the ball rolling.

I REFUSE TO EXCLUDE PLEASURE FROM EXERCISE

I have had a sedentary life for the past decade and a half. This makes it challenging to get into a routine that has physical exertion as an intrinsic part. Sarah Perry (2017) talks about it in her essay, "Body Pleasure." She points out that beginning a fitness routine also comes with the risk of entirely missing out on the pleasure zone of workouts, and I couldn't agree more. She advocates taking pleasure seriously and focusing on exercising for satisfaction. I would embrace it only if I could embrace it as slowly as I prefer and only at intensities that give me joy so I can retain my motivation and build a sustainable habit of working out.

I had to discover my threshold for keeping my workouts enjoyable—it varies from person to person. The risk of setting self-defeating standards is high because we end up perceiving exercise as "pain," and this needs to be deliberately cut out of the thought process. Ever since I began practicing yoga, I observed myself like never before, learning more about myself and garnering direct self-compassion and self-empathy instead of criticism and self-pity.

I was learning. From Jane and Sam, of course, but there were more teachers all around me. Sanders was finding his salvation in setting the tone for his workplace and Selena was in the process of finding her peace. Everybody's life presented lessons to learn from. I only had to keep my mind open.

8:00 p.m. a sense of balance

"Hey Mae, your phone's been ringing. Want me to bring it over?" Nolan asked as he walked past the kitchen.

"Later, dear. I'll call back; I am working."

"I thought you were exercising."

"Same thing."

CHAPTER 13

THE SCROLL

SCAN FOR AUDIO CHAPTER

I've listed my go-to poses and workouts here for you and anyone who wants to immerse themselves into a holistic health maintenance routine.

It is only the beginning—this collection will keep me going for years.

I want to continue learning and also hear about your progress. There will surely be additions as I move ahead in this quest. I hope you enjoy the meanderings as much as I do!

Love,
Maya

WHY BOTHER WITH WARM-UPS

I sit all day and want to be a diva with the perfect body. Getting into any intense and sustained body movement from a position of inertia would be like getting into the final stages of a lawsuit without dealing with preliminary rounds; you wouldn't be surprised if the whole case fell apart like a house of cards.

It makes sense to begin by mimicking the movements you plan to perform so that blood flow increases to those areas, your joints gear up for movement with lubrication, and your brain is prepared to get the right hormones flowing. It will allow you to understand what range of motion is pain-free for you.

In seated poses, the pelvis is placed on the chair, which can stress the joints connecting it to the legs and spine. This makes it particularly important to warm up the sacroiliac and hip joints sufficiently before twisting, bending, and turning.

Hours of sitting can stiffen the back, and starting with poses that stress them is a sure shot move to disaster. Thus, even a simple forward bend will pull at the ligaments if you don't prepare yourself with warm-ups. Getting up from your chair and moving around regularly is a good idea.

WHAT TO BE CAUTIOUS OF DURING CHAIR YOGA

My habit of wanting to see visible results in terms of the number of poses I could do would get me into trouble again and again. Body alignment instructions had to be dealt with carefully. I had to learn where to stretch and strengthen or risk hurting my knee or spraining my shoulders.

Jane told me I had to rely on myself to decide how much to push and that this discretion couldn't be outsourced even to a teacher.

"Over the years, I have seen countless instances of absolutely avoidable injuries. These invariably happen when the body sends signals and we ignore them. We tend to forget that yoga is a mind and body practice," she continued saying, "Use straps and blocks when you feel the need. Don't worry—you won't become dependent on them. Seated poses and exercises are as challenging as those done standing and moving around."

MAYA'S VIDEO LIBRARY

Complimentary Access

Video can play an important role in assisting the correct performance of yoga asanas. Therefore, with your purchase of The Maya Method you have lifetime access to Maya's video library.

Sign-Up for video access:

1.

   SCAN FOR VIDEO ACCESS

   or in your web brower enter:
   https://www.iaa.pub/maya-method-join

2. Click >'**Access All The Book's Videos**' button

3.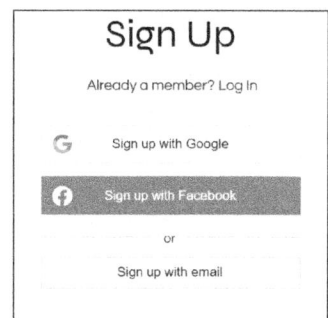

The videos have been specifically recorded to accompany Maya's Method and are an invaluable reference. Once signed-up simply visit www.iaa.pub

POSTURES HOW-TO

The Mountain Pose and Its Variations (Tadasana)

Mountain Posture on the Chair #1

SCAN FOR POSE AUDIO

How-to:

1. Find a chair without armrests and sit mindfully on the seat to feel the chair's texture. Bring awareness to your posture by first paying attention to your feet. Place them at hip-width distance for stability, with your toes pointing forward and well-grounded. Take your awareness to the soles of your feet. Even when you are in the office, try taking off your footwear. Leave your socks on if you must. This helps to feel grounded.

2. Your shins should be vertical to the ground and your knees should be pointing forward. If your feet can't comfortably reach the floor, use blocks under your feet to achieve the pose but ensure your knees don't rise above your thighs.

3. Flex your toes upward and back a few times to relax them while evenly distributing your body weight across your feet. Our sitting patterns, developed over many years, leaves us

with a less-than-ideal weight distribution on the back and legs. It's time to bring awareness to this.

4. Take your awareness upward to the leg muscles, groin, pelvis muscles, hips, spinal cord, and crown as if drawing energy from the ground to the crown. All muscles should be gently engaged, the sternum lifted, the navel tucked in, and the spine lengthened. As such, we fix the alignment of our bones, which has often gone haywire due to our daily habits.

5. Roll your shoulders back, open your chest, and place your arms on your thighs with your palms facing up or down. Watch out for any undue pressure as you progress. Your upper body needs a neutral position so your tailbone does not stick out while opening up your chest. This is the first step in correcting your posture and toning your muscles.

6. Relax your face, close your eyes, and lift the crown of your head by imagining a gentle force pulling it toward the sky. If you prefer keeping your eyes open, finding a spot to focus on helps.

7. Once your posture is taken care of, draw your attention to your breath. Focus on each breath that comes in and goes out. This is a sure-shot way to stop your mind from being distracted by thoughts. Feel your body and breath to calm your nervous system.

8. From this point on, you can move to warm-ups by rolling your neck, flexing your feet, raising your hands, and circling your shoulders to wake them up during long hours of sitting or working.

9. **Mountain Five-Pointed Pose** *(Utthita Tadasana)*: Stretching your arms wide at 45 degrees, with your fingers spread apart provides enough tension for your biceps and triceps.

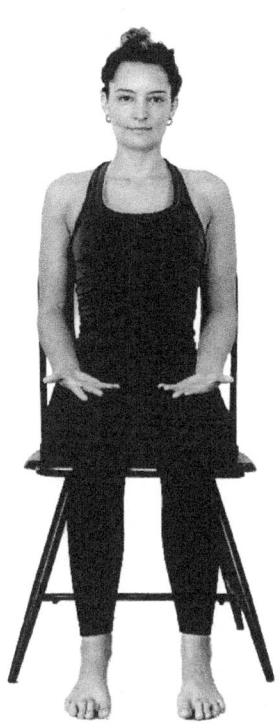

Mountain Pose With Side Stretch (Tiryaka Tadasana) #2

When the mountain pose described for the chair is adapted for a standing position, you get the classic tadasana. Once both poses are under your belt, look for some deeper stretches.

Performing the side stretch pose after drinking two glasses of warm water early in the morning is a time-tested method to clear the intestines and lose weight.

SCAN FOR POSE AUDIO

How-to:

1. Take the seated mountain stance, gently raise both arms from the sides, and interlock your fingers above the crown of your head.

2. Turn your wrists so your palms face the sky. Hold this position for a few breaths until you feel the stretch through your sides.

3. Keeping your fingers firmly interlocked, bend your waist to the right without bending your elbows.

4. Hold this position and repeat on the opposite side.

CHAIR YOGA FOR WEIGHT LOSS

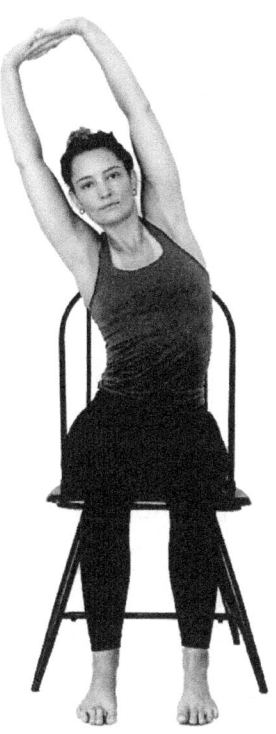

Back Bound Mountain Pose (Baddha Hasta Tadasana) #3

SCAN FOR POSE AUDIO

How-to:

1. Assume the upright position standing on the yoga mat. Once you have brought your awareness to your entire body and connected to your breath, prepare for this deep hand stretch.

2. Take your arms behind you, without raising them, and interlock your fingers next to your glutes with your palms facing downward.

3. Gently raise your arms away from your body without bending your elbows. Try to raise them as much as possible. This may not come easy initially, so do not fret.

4. Simultaneously tilt your head backward gently so that you face the sky. Hold this position for a few breaths before releasing your hands and returning to an upright position.

This is a good upper arm and belly stretching pose that will improve your overall posture in the long run.

CHAIR YOGA FOR WEIGHT LOSS

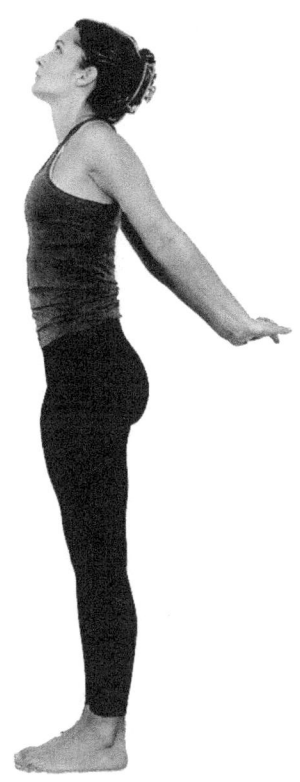

The Raised Hand Pose and Its Variations (Urdhava Hastasana)

Raised Hands Pose #4

SCAN FOR POSE AUDIO

How-to:

1. Assume the standing mountain posture with all the attention it deserves, engaging your muscles from head to toe as per the method elaborated.

2. Pay attention to your arms and open up your palms so your wrists rotate outward. Raise your hands from your sides by stretching them well so that your fingers point to the ceiling. Clasp your palms together in a prayer position if you feel flexible enough. Otherwise, they can remain parallel to each other.

3. You will need to take time to check your posture at this point. The hand raise must result in your rib cage lifting equally from all sides.

4. Keep your sternum vertical (as if it needs to point to your pelvis), navel tucked in, and tailbone pushed downward. This will also ensure that your shoulder blades are pushed down.

5. Keep your arms active by pushing your elbows up. Then stretch moving upward. You will notice that your fingers will also be engaged.

6. Your gaze should follow your palms with your neck gently stretched upward. Hold the position for a few relaxed breaths, then return back to the mountain posture.

7. While the mountain posture gives you the feeling of being rooted to the earth, this posture will add a layer of an opposing force toward the sky. Stay in this posture to soak in the feeling of release, with the energy flowing upward through your spine and arms, all while feeling the stability of being rooted.

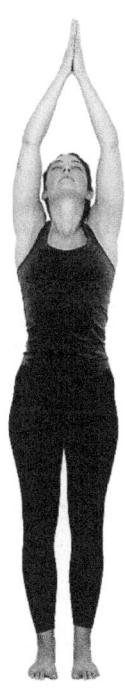

Crescent Moon on the Chair
(Parsva Urdhva Hastasana) #5

SCAN FOR POSE AUDIO

How-to:

1. Sit straight on the chair while keeping your legs slightly apart.

2. With your gaze directed in front, extend both arms to the side and bring them together on top of the crown of your head in the prayer position. Close your eyes as you do so. Breathe in deeply, and feel your spine lengthen as you lift your rib cage equally from all sides.

3. Gently bend to the right to provide your left rib cage with a nice, relaxed stretch while holding your breath. Hold for four counts and breathe out while straightening up again. You will realize that sustaining this pose needs good core strength.

4. Bring your hands down, relax, and open your eyes. Feel the sensations of your body and repeat on the left side. The raised-hand poses can be done seated or standing with equal effect.

CHAIR YOGA FOR WEIGHT LOSS

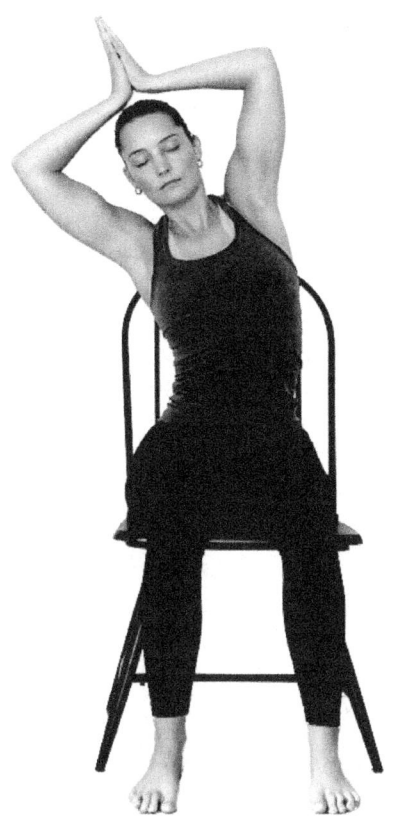

The Tree Pose (Vrikshasana)

The Standing Tree Pose #6

SCAN FOR POSE AUDIO

How-to:

1. This pose is performed by first assuming the mountain pose. Make sure to warm up by stretching your upper body gently if this is the first pose you are practicing.

2. From the upright position, begin by raising the heel of your right foot to get the feel of your body weight shifting from both legs to the left leg.

3. Slowly raise your right leg and rest it on the side of your left leg, touching your inner thigh, or the side of your shin, while avoiding your knee joint. Initially, you may need to lift your leg with your hands and place your foot in position.

4. Keep your left foot firmly grounded by ensuring your ankle bone is firm, calf muscles and quadriceps are engaged, and hip bones are aligned with your upper body. Take time to find your balance after the initial feeling of instability. This would mean closely observing the alignment of your whole body, especially ensuring that you keep your navel tucked in and tailbone pointing down instead of jutting backward.

5. Once you feel stable enough, raise both hands by your sides and extend them upward into a prayer position above the crown of your head. If that seems too difficult, keep your arms parallel to each other. You could even do a variation with your hands spread out in a V-shape.

6. Hold the pose with your eyes open and gaze straight ahead to maintain your balance for several seconds to feel its effect on every part of your body. With practice, you will feel grace and serenity.

7. Release by bringing your leg down gently and getting back into the upright position. Repeat on the opposite side.

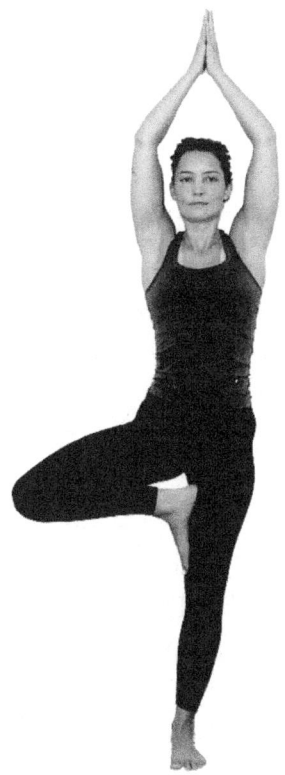

The Cat-Cow Pose (Marjaryasana-Bitilasana)

The Cat-Cow Stretch on the Floor #7

When done efficiently, this pose will give you immediate relief from lower back pain resulting from prolonged sitting or standing sessions. Since our spines do not get to move enough, stiffness sets in much to our discomfort. The cat-cow pose also benefits digestion and has a calming effect on the mind.

SCAN FOR POSE AUDIO

How-to:

1. Get down on all fours on the yoga mat with your palms, knees, and toes supporting your body weight. Take time to align your body and ensure your shoulders are directly above your wrists and your knees are directly under your hip bones.

2. Inhale here.

3. Exhale deeply as you tuck your tailbone, push the floor away arching your back and separate your shoulder blades. Keep your head down and try to bring your gaze to your navel as you get into a position resembling a cat.

4. Next, inhale and relax the arch by bringing your belly down and tilting your pelvis forward. Pull your head back to look upwards, as you get into a position resembling a cow.

5. Ensure that your spine moves up and down, not front and back. Most people tend to swing their bodies; avoid doing that. Notice that your shoulder blades will move apart in the cat pose and come together in the cow pose. Alternate at least a dozen times with smooth movements to flex your spine.

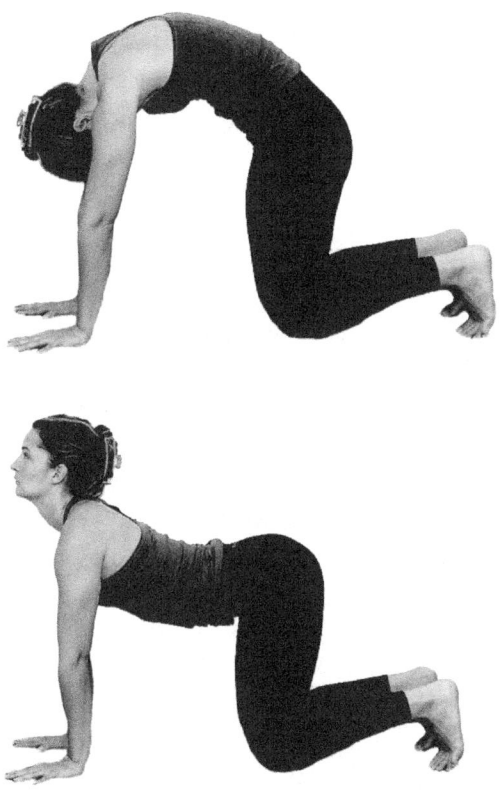

Chair Cat-Cow (Marjaryasana-Bitilasana) #8

SCAN FOR POSE AUDIO

How-to:

1. Sit upright toward the front edge of your chair with your feet placed firmly on the ground. Bring your hands onto your knees with your palms facing down. This will help you gently grasp your knees to keep your movement rhythmic.

2. Lift your chest while inhaling and round your back to exhale. This pattern will help you breathe comfortably.

3. The cat pose is achieved by exhaling and pushing your shoulders forward, rounding your upper back to get your spinal cord into an arch, lowering your head to drop your chin on your chest, and drawing your abdominal muscles in. The cow pose is achieved by inhaling and pushing your chest and spine forward, bringing your shoulders down, raising your head, bringing your shoulder blades together, and keeping your core engaged.

CHAIR YOGA FOR WEIGHT LOSS

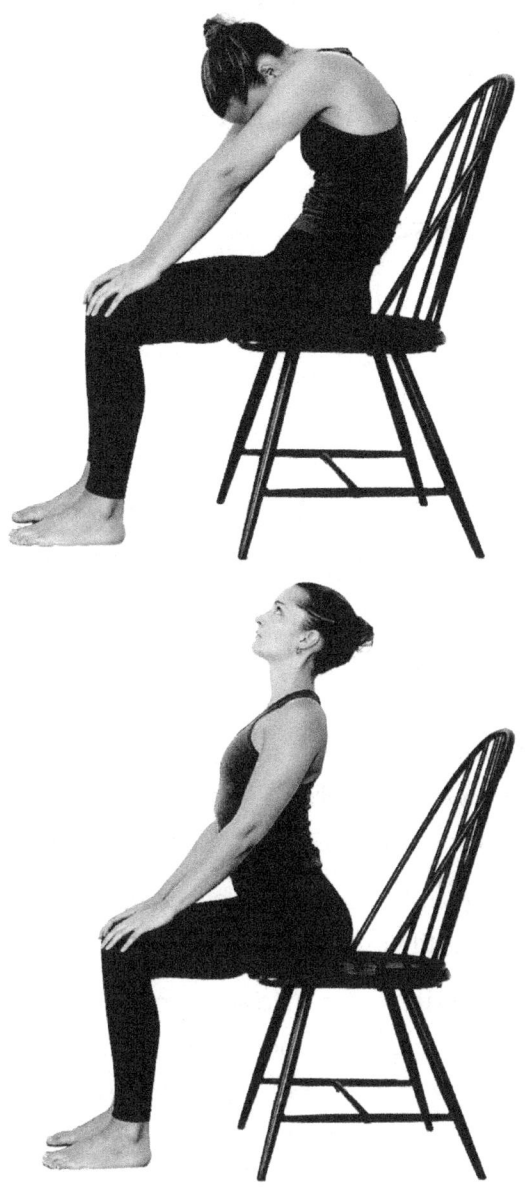

The Forward Fold Pose and Its Variations (Uttanasana)

Half Forward-Fold (Ardha Uttanasana) #9

SCAN FOR POSE AUDIO

How-to:

1. The idea is to learn to keep your back flat while bending. Stand straight on the mat in the mountain pose. Keep your legs straight, exhale, bend forward, and let your arms rest on your shinbones.

2. Your spine should be straight, your navel pulled in, your chest open with your shoulders rolled back, and your head held such that your gaze rests slightly ahead.

3. While your legs should be straight, you can slightly bend your knees until you get more flexible.

4. Hold this position for a few seconds and inhale while returning to the upright position. Giving yourself a gentle backward stretch helps neutralize the intense forward fold.

CHAIR YOGA FOR WEIGHT LOSS

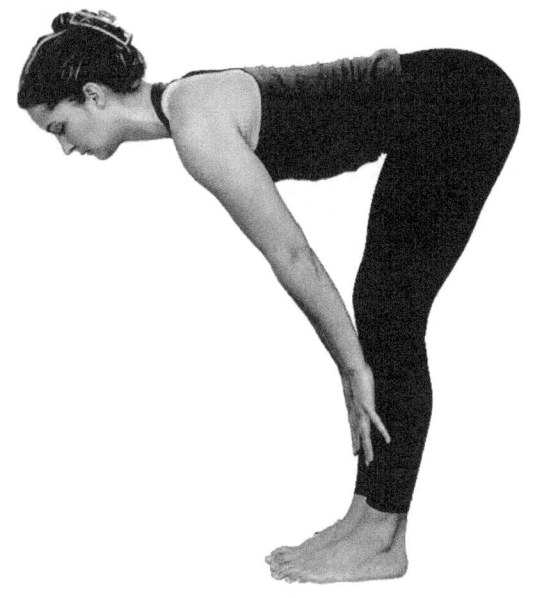

Forward Fold Pose on the Chair (Uttanasana) #10

SCAN FOR POSE AUDIO

How-to:

1. Sit toward the front of the seat and keep your legs hip-width apart.

2. Inhale while raising both hands, exhale, and bend forward to rest your chest on your thighs.

3. Bring your hands to the sides of your feet and try to place your palms on the ground. Bend as much as you comfortably can. It may be a good idea to place blocks at your feet so your palms can rest on them for initial practice.

4. Get back upright while raising your hands and rest. Repeat a few times to improve flexibility.

CHAIR YOGA FOR WEIGHT LOSS

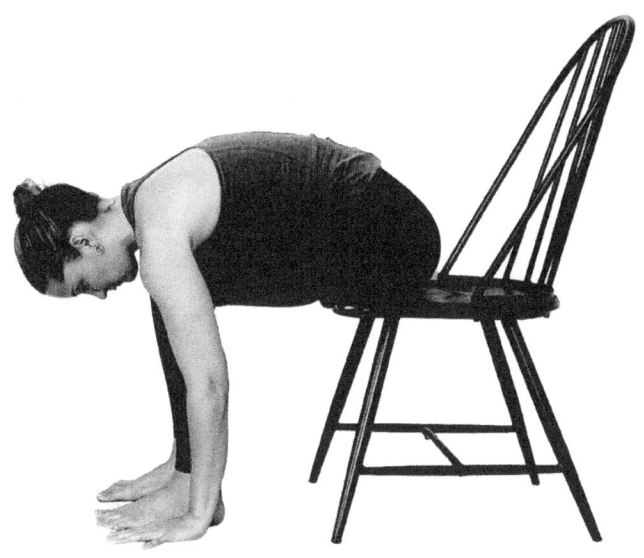

Standing Forward Fold (Uttanasana) #11

This intermediate-level pose should only be attempted once you gain mastery over the anatomy of yogic movements and your body has achieved the necessary strength and flexibility.

SCAN FOR POSE AUDIO

How-to:

1. Stand upright with your feet hip-width apart. To begin the forward fold, you will need to bend from your hip crease. Failure to do so will result in a stooped upper back, which would be counterproductive to the pose.

2. With your hands at your hip crease, begin to fold your upper body wholly without changing the alignment of your spine, chest, or shoulders. Fold it over your legs much like you would fold a towel.

3. Your hamstrings will let you know the extent to which you can bend.

4. As you bend, slide your palms down from your knees to your toes and rest them as far down your legs as possible. The goal is to place them by the side of your feet or even further behind. Placing them in front will result in a forward swing; we do not want that.

5. The perfect posture is an intense bend that will have your legs straightened, hips and tailbone lifted, your chest touching your knees, and the crown of your head facing the ground, making you feel balanced and calm. Mastering this will take weeks but is well worth the effort.

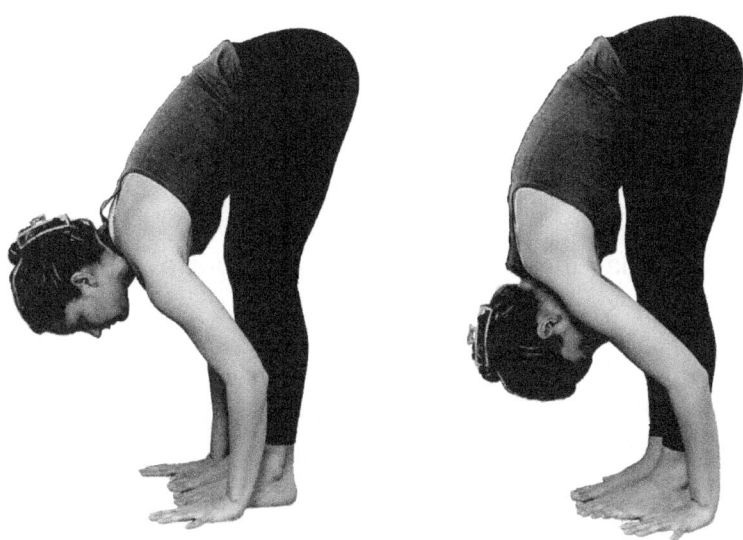

The Crescent Lunge (Anjaneyasana) #12

This pose is achieved by kneeling behind a chair and using the backrest to maintain balance as you perform a low lunge. It especially helps open up your hip joints.

 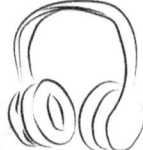

SCAN FOR POSE AUDIO

How-to:

1. Place a chair in front of you, about a foot away. Slightly bend from your waist to hold both sides of the backrest around the halfway point.

2. Holding firm, allow your right leg to stretch backward as you kneel on the floor. Place your left leg at a right angle. Hold the lunge for 10 counts while maintaining balance. You will notice your body weight on both metatarsals.

3. Gently return to the standing position and repeat with your left leg. As you get better with the lunges, you can add variations by raising your arms in the lunge position and twisting your upper body.

CHAIR YOGA FOR WEIGHT LOSS

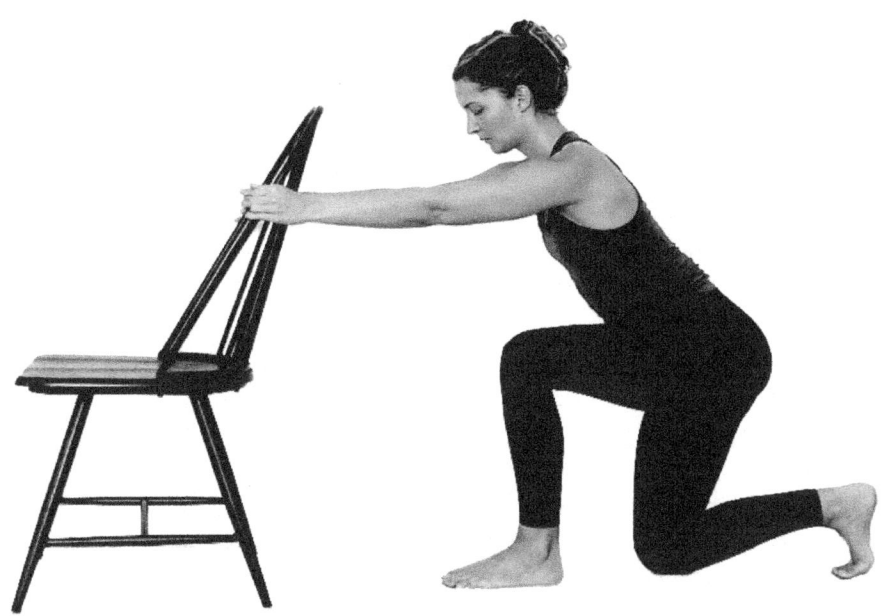

Happy Baby Pose (Upavistha Ardha Ananda Balasana) #13

SCAN FOR POSE AUDIO

How-to:

1. From the seated mountain pose, lift your right leg and place your foot on the chair seat. Bring your thighs close to your chest and gently lift your foot with the help of your right hand so your calf is parallel to the ground. Hold this position for 10 counts and repeat on the opposite side.
2. Your thigh should remain close to your upper body. Focus on your spine to maintain a vertical pose.
3. This pose is a great way to stretch your hamstrings and hips. It also works well to release tension in your shoulders.

CHAIR YOGA FOR WEIGHT LOSS

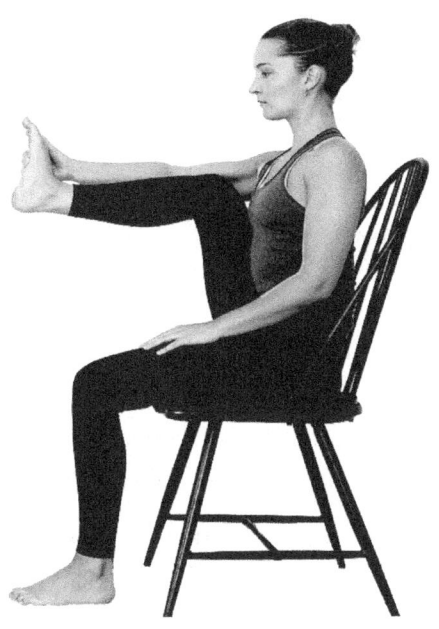

Head to Knee Pose (Parivrtta Janu Sirsasana) #14

SCAN FOR POSE AUDIO

How-to:

1. From the upright position, lift your right leg to rest on the seat with your foot touching your inner left thigh.

2. Stretch your left leg toward the side of the chair. Take your time to achieve balance and adjust your waist to position your left leg stably on the ground.

3. Place your left arm across your tummy, gently raise your right arm, and bend your waist upward, toward the left. Keep your gaze to the right as you bend and ensure your left leg remains rooted on the floor. Hold for 10 counts and repeat on the opposite side.

4. Feel your ribs opening up as you bend; it is so relaxing. This pose can be challenging if your lower back and thigh muscles are not yet flexible. Do not force the position. Take your time to achieve the perfect pose.

CHAIR YOGA FOR WEIGHT LOSS

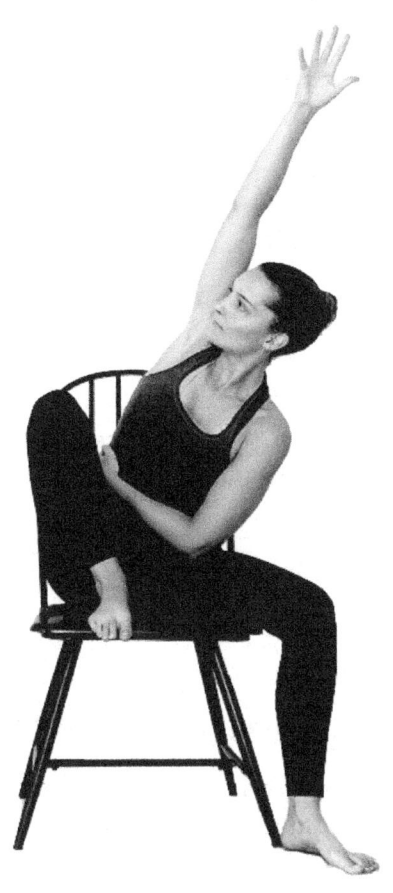

Marichi Pose (Marichyasana) #15

SCAN FOR POSE AUDIO

How-to:

1. From the upright position, move yourself to the front edge of your chair. Lift your right leg, and place your foot on the chair seat. Extend your left leg to the side of the chair. Hold this position and pay attention to your entire body to check for any discomfort.

2. Now place your right elbow on your inner right knee with your fingers pointing upward. Take your left hand back to hold the backrest.

3. Breathe in as you stabilize the pose and gently turn your waist to the side of your extended leg. Hold the position for 10 counts and repeat on the opposite side.

4. The rotation of your upper body and pelvis in opposite directions benefits your body's flexibility as long as your movements are attentive and gentle.

CHAIR YOGA FOR WEIGHT LOSS

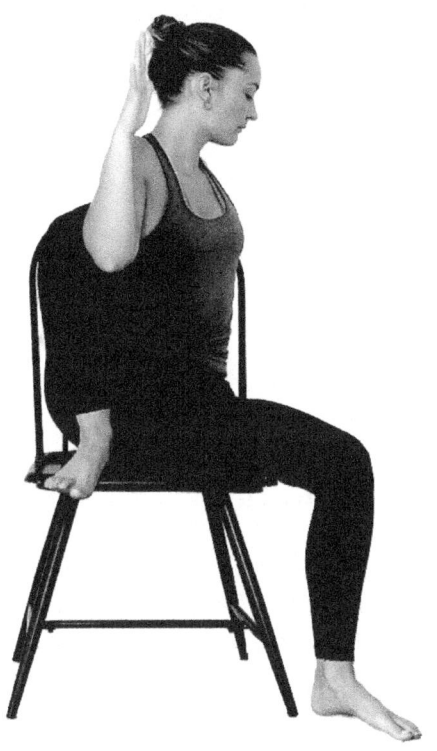

Sun Salutation (Suryanamaskar) #16

SCAN FOR POSE AUDIO

How-to:

1. Sit upright with your hands folded in a prayer position before your chest. Inhale and exhale once to bring your focus to the pose.

2. Inhale and raise both arms, arching your back to bend slightly backward Feel the stretch of your rib cage and spine. Hold the position as you hold your breath for a few seconds.

3. Exhale and come to the fold-forward position. Your chest should rest on your lap and your palms should touch the ground.

4. Inhale and lift your upper body back to an upright position. As you do so, sweep your right leg up by supporting your thighs from below with both hands. Bring your foot to the chair seat level to feel your hamstring stretch.

5. Bend your upper body to touch your nose to your right knee. Exhale and release your leg back gently to the ground.

6. Inhale and raise your hands to repeat with your left foot raised this time.

 This sequence can be repeated as many times as you can for a complete body warm-up.

CHAIR YOGA FOR WEIGHT LOSS

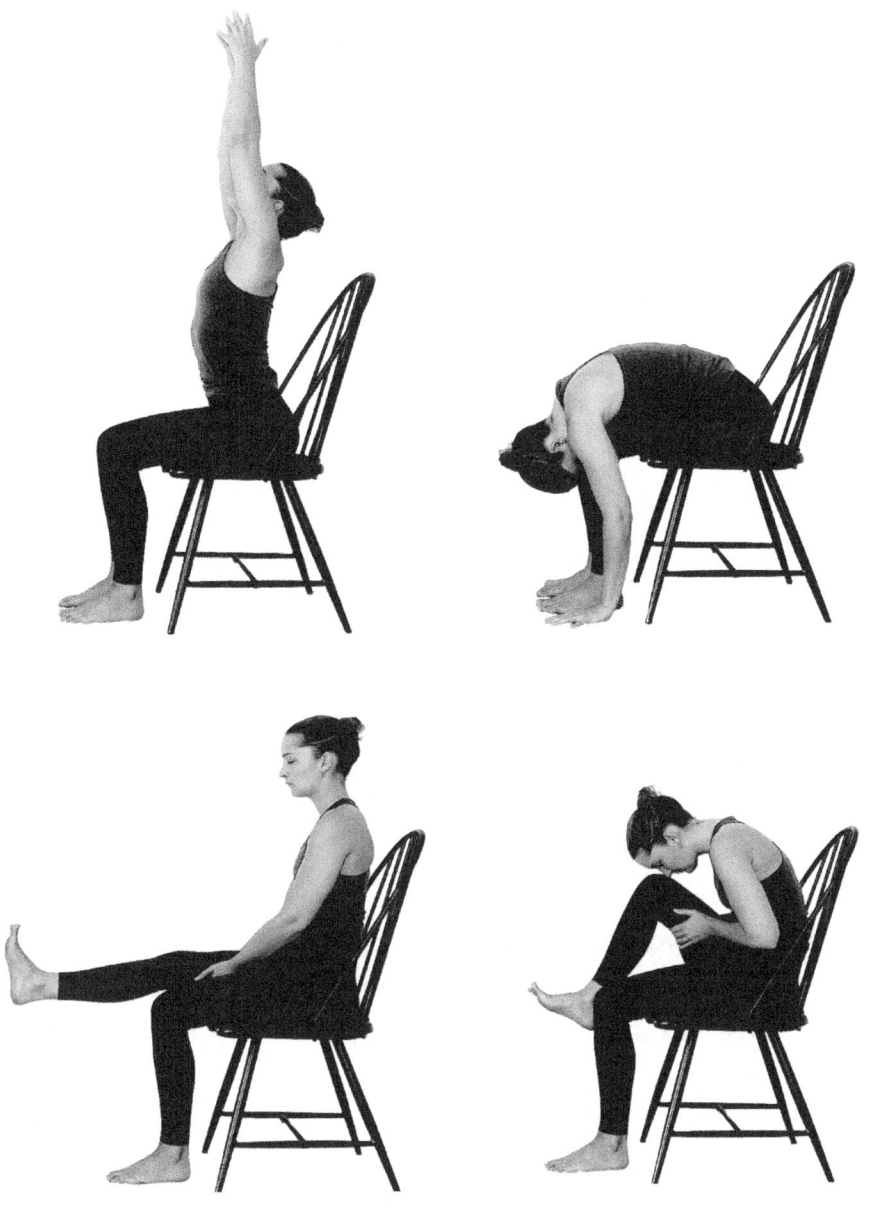

Cobra Pose (Bhujangasana) #17

SCAN FOR POSE AUDIO

How-to:

1. Sit upright toward the front of the chair with your spine extended.

2. Take both arms behind you and hold the edge of the seat so you feel a stretch in your biceps. Inhale and bend your head back gently to open your chest muscles. Your shoulder blades should come together.

3. Note any strain in the neck area. If you feel discomfort, release the pose and do some neck rotation warm-ups.

4. Once you can hold the backward bend position comfortably, look upward, exhale, and hold the position, feeling the stretch in your chest and midriff. Inhale and exhale for 10 counts as you feel the energy flow in your throat and upper body. Relax and get back to an upright position without causing any jerks to the neck.

CHAIR YOGA FOR WEIGHT LOSS

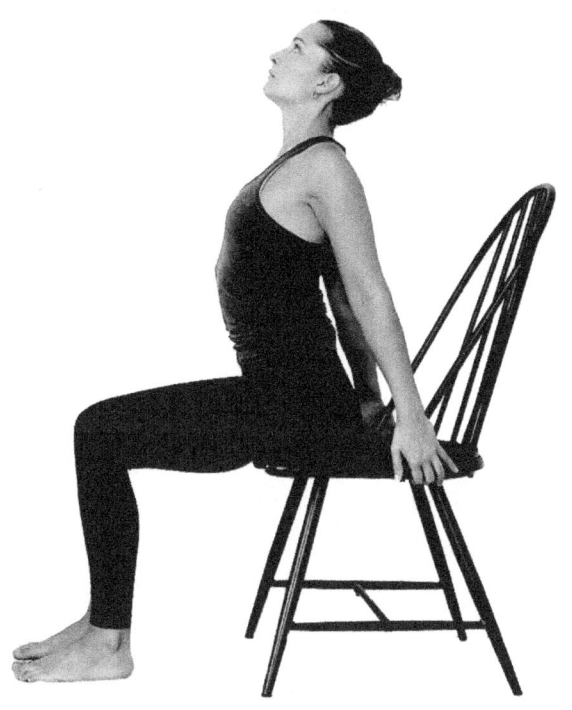

Dolphin Pose (Ardha Pincha Mayurasana) #18

SCAN FOR POSE AUDIO

How-to:

1. Kneel on the yoga mat and bend forward to place your elbows and forearms on the mat. Interlock your fingers to get your pose well-balanced. Take a few deep breaths to relax.

2. Curl back your toes so that your heels face upward. Your thighs should be perpendicular to the ground, and you should be facing the ground.

3. Exhale and lift your knees and hips so your body resembles an inverted V. It is somewhat similar to the downward dog pose except your elbows are placed firmly on the floor.

4. Your shoulder blades have to hold firm. Ensure to keep your shoulders away from your ears.

5. Hold the position for about five breaths while adjusting your feet so that your weight is on your metatarsals and your heels nearly touch the ground.

6. To get out of the pose, bring down your knees, relax your feet, and straighten up. It's best to get into the child's pose to relax before you get off the floor.

CHAIR YOGA FOR WEIGHT LOSS

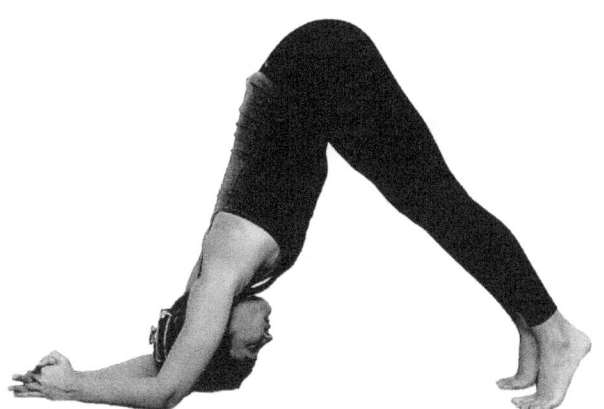

Hand-to-Toes (Hasta Padangusthasana) #19

This pose provides deep hamstring stretching. It also tests the flexibility of your upper back.

SCAN FOR POSE AUDIO

How-to:

1. From the upright position, extend your right leg toward the front and keep your toes pointing upward. You will notice that your glutes will slide toward the front edge of the chair for better balance.

2. Bend your upper body from your hips toward your right thigh by keeping your back straight.

3. Keeping your left palm on your thigh, extend your right hand toward your big toe and grasp it with your thumb and pointer finger. Make sure your knees don't bend. Your arm and leg will appear to be in parallel lines, meeting at the toes. Hold this position for five counts.

4. Keep your gaze to the front and take time to feel the sensations. The hip bend and hamstring stretch will be an experience in itself. Repeat on the left side.

CHAIR YOGA FOR WEIGHT LOSS

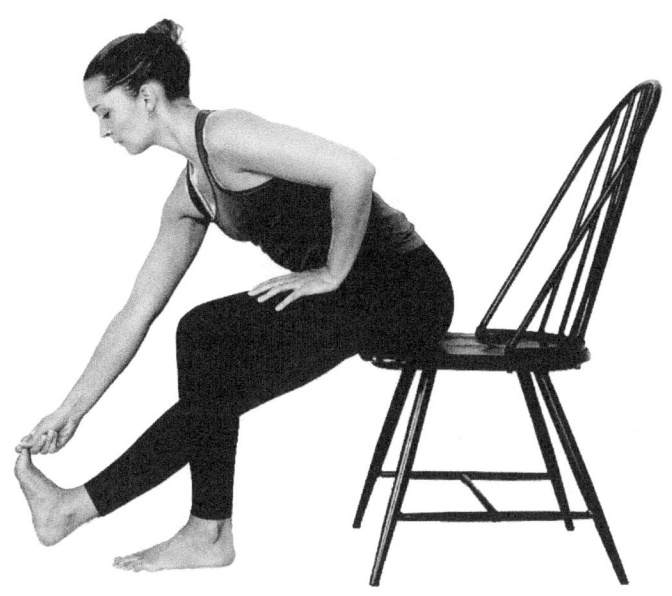

Hand-to-Toes Variation With Strap #20

SCAN FOR POSE AUDIO

How-to:

1. Assume the mountain pose on the chair and relax with a few rounds of inhalation and exhalation.

2. Loop your yoga strap (or a rolled-up towel) around your right foot and hold the other end, adjusting its length to tighten it to the same length as your leg.

3. Inhale and pull the strap while keeping your hips and lower back snug on the chair until your leg is raised to about knee height. Your left leg must be firmly on the ground for good balance.

4. Ensure your back is straight and your chest and shoulders are opened up well. Hold this position for six to eight counts while breathing deeply. Keeping the strap pulled toward your body will help support your leg for a longer time. This is great for the hamstrings and calf muscles.

5. To release, bring your leg down by releasing the strap gently while firmly gripping it with your hands. Remove the strap to repeat with the left leg. This pose provides the necessary blood circulation during long hours at work.

CHAIR YOGA FOR WEIGHT LOSS

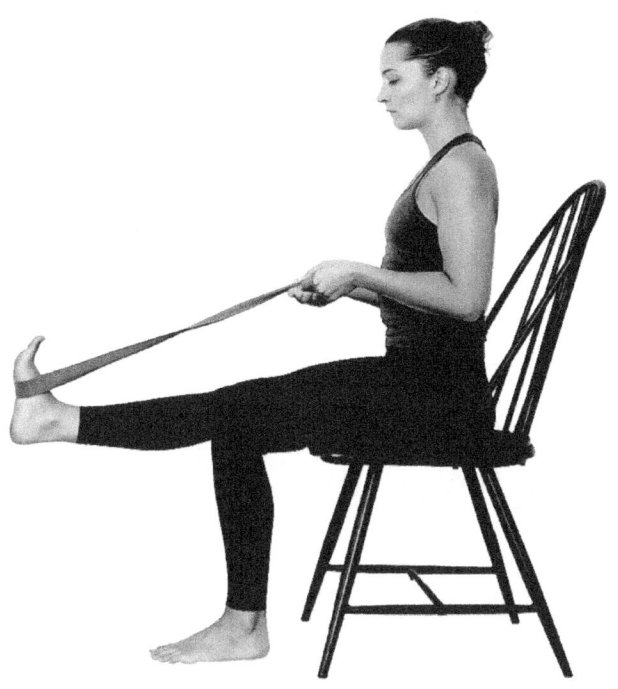

Easy Pose (Sukhasana) #21

This pose enables you to look within and harmonize your physical and emotional selves. Be warned the name is deceptive as it is going to test your core strength.

If you feel unstable performing the Easy Pose on a chair, you can sit on the floor if your mobility permits.

SCAN FOR POSE AUDIO

How-to:

1. Assume the mountain pose, fold one or both legs onto the seat of the chair.
2. With shoulders open and elbows up to chest level, assume a prayer stance with your palms together at the base of your sternum.
3. Inhale and exhale intentionally and keep moving your attention to the pelvis to make sure there is proper weight distribution and then to the upper body periodically.
4. Hold the position for 1 minute. Yes, it will be challenging at first to maintain this position for a full 60 seconds.

CHAIR YOGA FOR WEIGHT LOSS

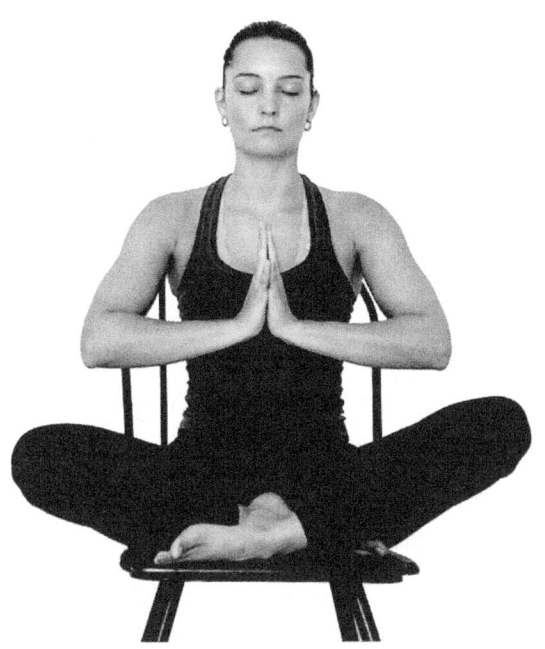

Lion Pose (Simhasana) #22

SCAN FOR POSE AUDIO

How-to:

1. Assume the mountain pose to bring your attention to the present. You can either assume the cross-legged pose on the floor or remain in the mountain pose on the chair to proceed through this pose.

2. Spread your fingers wide apart with your palms facing downward. Place your palms firmly on your knees and feel your shoulder blades pressing on your back as you do so.

3. As you inhale deeply, open your mouth and stick your tongue out so it points to your chin. Notice that you'll inhale through your nose and mouth at this point.

4. Keep your eyes open, either directing your gaze toward your nose or upward toward the center of your eyebrows. Hold your breath for a couple of seconds. Exhale long through your throat with a "ha" sound. Hold this open-mouth position comfortably for about six seconds.

5. Close your mouth to inhale and exhale normally for one count each and repeat the pose five to six times. Make sure you don't strain your mouth. Ensure gentle movements and maintain a proper posture.

Practicing the lion pose keeps the platysma firm. The platysma is a broad muscle situated in the neck region below the chin. When the muscles and skin are not toned, it pulls down the corners of the mouth resulting in the "turkey neck" and causing your face to wrinkle as you age.

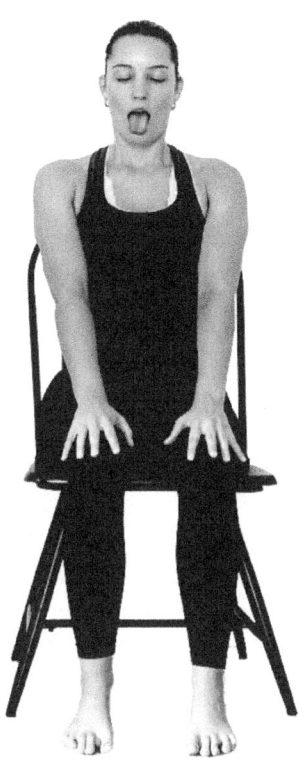

Chin Lock Pose (Jalandhara Bandha) #23

SCAN FOR POSE AUDIO

How-to:

1. Either assume the mountain or easy pose and begin by inhaling deeply. Hold your breath and move your chin down toward your chest. Simultaneously, lift your sternum and chest upward to "lock" your windpipe.
2. Notice your shoulders moving inward. You will feel your chest open up since you have inhaled air.
3. Hold your breath in this position for as long as you feel comfortable.
4. Raise your chin back to position while exhaling deeply.
5. Relax and breathe normally. This can be repeated three to four times in one sitting.

This exercise not only tones your facial muscles but also improves concentration and your ability to hold your breath.

CHAIR YOGA FOR WEIGHT LOSS

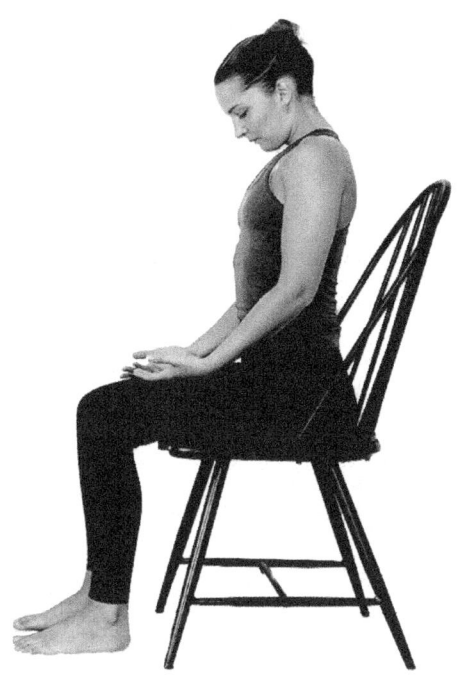

The Downward Dog Pose and Its Variations

Downward Dog on the Chair (Adho Mukha Svanasana) #24

This variation allows you to get the benefit of the pose while being seated on the chair and not having to be on the ground.

SCAN FOR POSE AUDIO

How-to:

1. Move your glutes toward the front edge of the chair. Sit upright with your spine lengthened.

2. Stretch both your legs forward. Keep them slightly wide with your toes facing upward. Take your time to gently pull your toes toward you. You will feel your ankles and hamstrings stretching. At this point, bring your attention to your lower spine and stretch it upward to prevent any slouching.

3. Now, gently raise both your arms forward and keep them raised at a 45-degree angle. Bend forward as if to push an imaginary wall. Hold this position for about 20 seconds to allow resistance to build up and feel your arm muscles fire up.

4. Thrusting your legs and arms forward will lengthen your entire back, starting from the arches of your feet to the crown of your head, while toning your arm muscles.

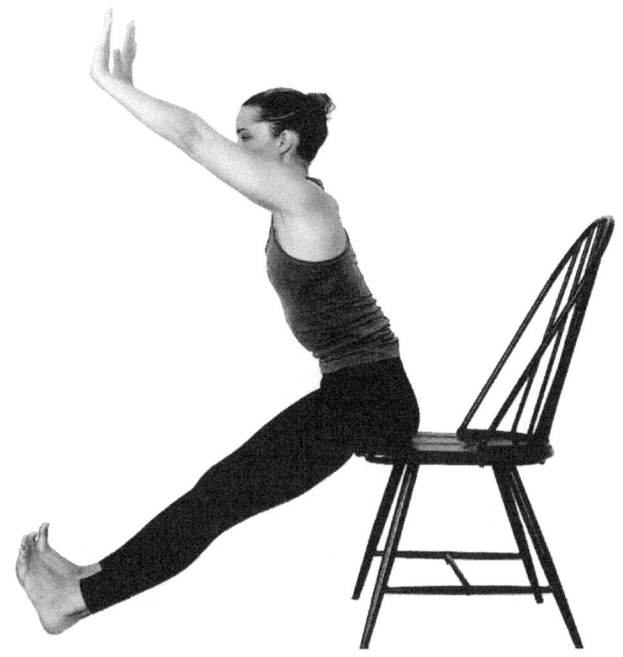

Wide-Legged Downward Dog Pose (Prasarita Adho Mukha Svanasana) #25

This prone posture is achieved by getting off the chair and using it to support your upper body.

SCAN FOR POSE AUDIO

How-to:

1. Face your chair and stand about a foot away from it. Keep your feet hip-width apart for stability.

2. Inhale, raise your hands, bend forward, and place your palms on the chair seat. At this point, it is important to bring your attention to your weight distribution. Retain strength at your core and pelvic muscles by keeping them taut so your shoulders and neck are protected from undue strain.

3. Your arms should maintain a shoulder-width distance on the chair. Keep your head down so that you can gaze at your feet. Take some deep breaths while checking your overall comfort.

4. Walk back two to three steps keeping your feet hip-width apart for a good muscle stretch. The angle should be such that you begin to feel your hamstrings pull gently.

5. Hold this position for six to eight breaths to feel calm as the blood flow improves in your upper body. To release, walk forward and lift your arms off the chair to return to an upright position.

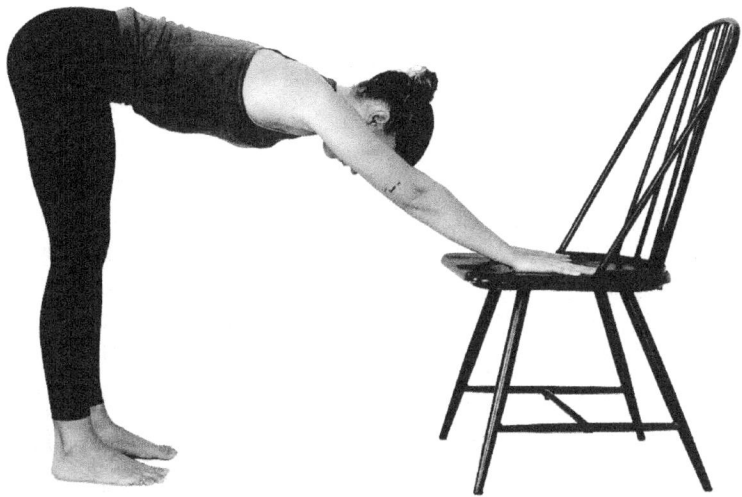

The Downward Dog on the Floor (Adho Mukha Svanasana) #26

SCAN FOR POSE AUDIO

How-to:

1. Get down on all fours on the mat by bending your knees to touch the floor and fully extending your arms with your palms resting down and fingers spread out.

2. Your toes will point down with your heels facing the ceiling. Keep your feet hip-width apart. Thrust your tailbone up and allow your spine to curve slightly so your back resembles a tabletop while bringing your awareness to all the muscles involved. The cat-cow pose will help relax your spine before you come to straighten it with your gaze downward.

3. Lift your hips to form a triangle. Keep your head down with your gaze on your toes. Your ears should be in alignment with your biceps. Keep your feet flat on the floor to maximize the benefits of this stretch. If your heels initially tend to lift slightly off the floor, that's okay. Stretching your hamstrings before attempting this pose and practicing regularly will help keep your heels grounded.

4. Tighten your core muscles by pulling your navel in to keep your strength in the midsection. Maintain this pose for a

few breaths. Note any undue pressure on your wrists and shoulders. As you get deeper into the practice, you will learn to feel completely calm in the pose as if it were a resting position.

5. Release the pose by lifting your heels, dropping your knees onto the ground, and sitting upright.

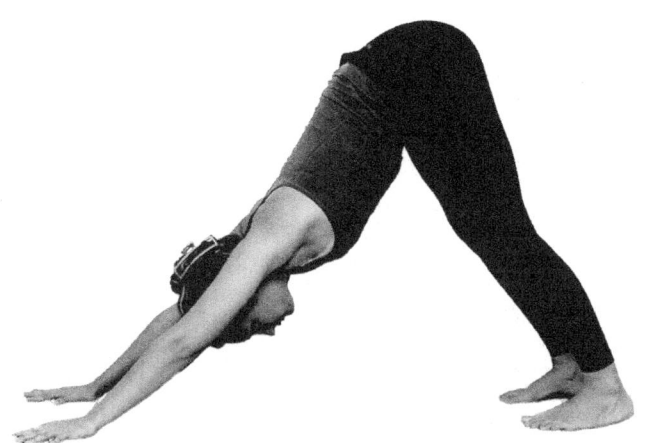

Three-Legged Downward Dog (Tri Pada Adho Mukha Svanasana) #27

This is an intense hip-opening pose of intermediate difficulty and should be done after the initial poses are mastered.

SCAN FOR POSE AUDIO

How-to:

1. Once you assume the downward dog position on the floor, check if your hips are lifted up well enough. Your arms will feel some load when your leg goes up.
2. Check the alignment of your shoulders with your hips.
3. Your hips need to be squared, not twisted to the side. This will allow you to lift your leg straight up without wobbling.
4. Extend your right leg back and lift it as much as you can. Keep your toes spread, push your heels backwards, and ensure your knee faces downward.
5. Your shoulders or arms should not cave in at any point.
6. Hold this position for six to eight breaths and repeat on the opposite side.

CHAIR YOGA FOR WEIGHT LOSS

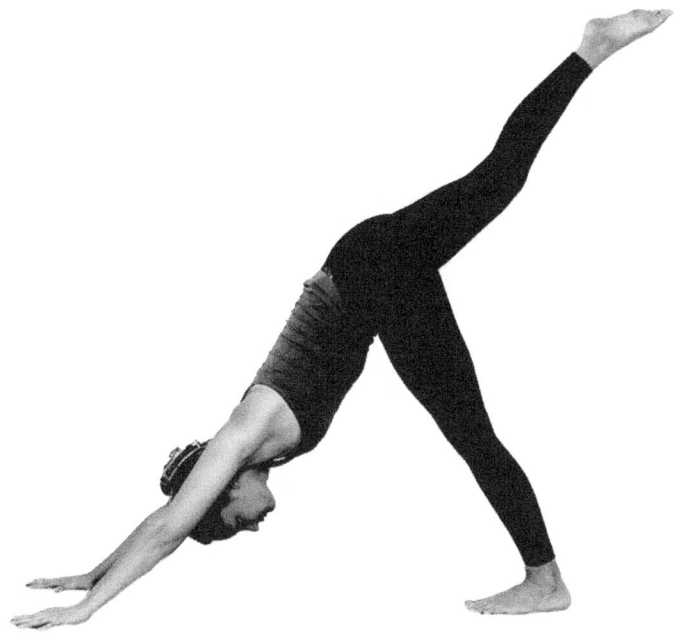

The Warrior Pose and Its Variations

The Warrior 1 Pose (Virabhadrasana 1) #28

Getting into the warrior pose through the downward dog pose is a good idea.

SCAN FOR POSE AUDIO

How-to:

1. From the downward dog, get into the high lunge position by taking your right leg forward to place your foot between your resting palms with your leg at a 90-degree angle. Your right knee should be stacked over your ankle. Rest your left foot down at 45 degrees.

2. Lift your upper body so it's vertical to the ground. Simultaneously raise both your arms, passing them by the side of your ears, and extend them above the crown of your head in the prayer position. This can be hard; you will need regular practice.

3. You will now be in a high lunge position with your front leg at a right angle and your back leg stretched well. Keep your hips square. Lower your hip slightly for stability. You will begin to feel a burn in your quads and a stretch in your entire body—that's good.

4. Extend your hands backward by arching your chest and letting your gaze follow your arms. Your shoulders should not be pushed backward, which is a common tendency. Hold this position with relaxed breathing for 10–12 seconds and repeat with the opposite leg. Return to the downward dog pose; this time, bring your left foot forward.

Your ability to sustain the pose will improve with time as your quads and arms get stronger. Don't push through the pain. It's best to increase your range of motion gradually.

You can recreate the full pose on the chair:

How-to:

1. Begin by sitting toward the front edge of the chair with your legs spread on the sides.
2. Turn your upper body to the right while turning and extending your arms upward.
3. Stretch your left leg back with your heel resting on the floor at 45 degrees. Keep your right leg at a right angle by turning your right foot outward. Reach both hands overhead. Voila! You have your pose.

CHAIR YOGA FOR WEIGHT LOSS

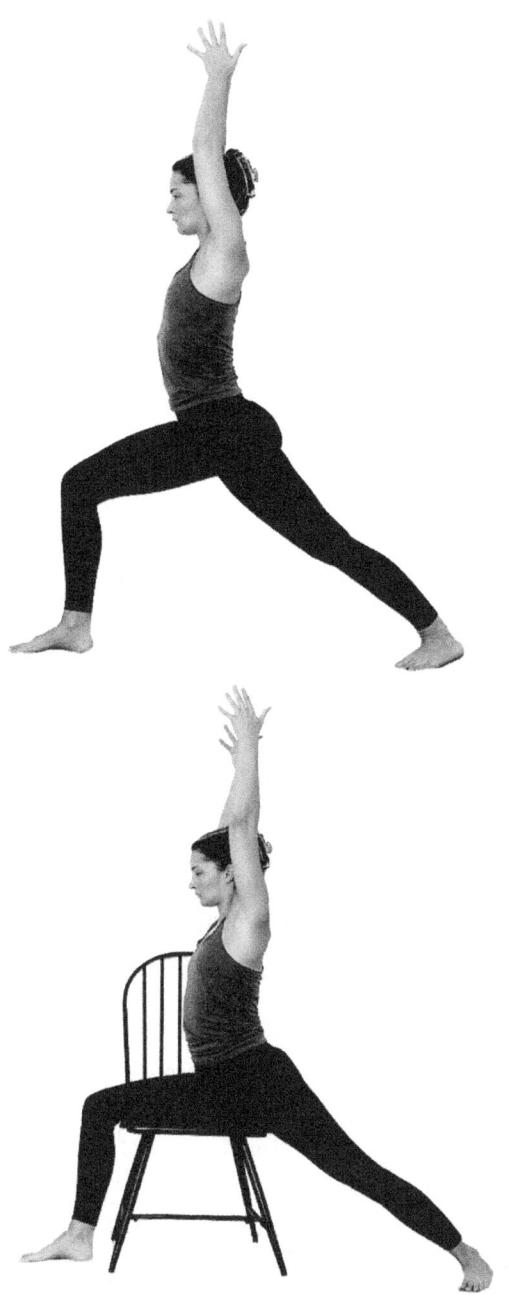

The Warrior 2 Pose (Virabhadrasana 2) #29

SCAN FOR POSE AUDIO

How-to:

1. This pose begins the same way as the Warrior 1 pose. Once you get into the high lunge position, rotate your back foot to 90 degrees, allowing your hips to open to the front of the chair. Bring your arms down to the height of your shoulders and spread them straight.

2. Your right hand should be parallel to your right thigh with your fingers pointing forward. Your left hand should be stretched behind, following your left leg. Keep your gaze over your front hand.

3. Maintain your balance by grounding the big toe of your right leg and the heel of your left leg. Stay in this position for 10–12 seconds and repeat on the opposite side.

4. Keeping your legs in two different directions is indeed tough and a good challenge to live up to.

CHAIR YOGA FOR WEIGHT LOSS

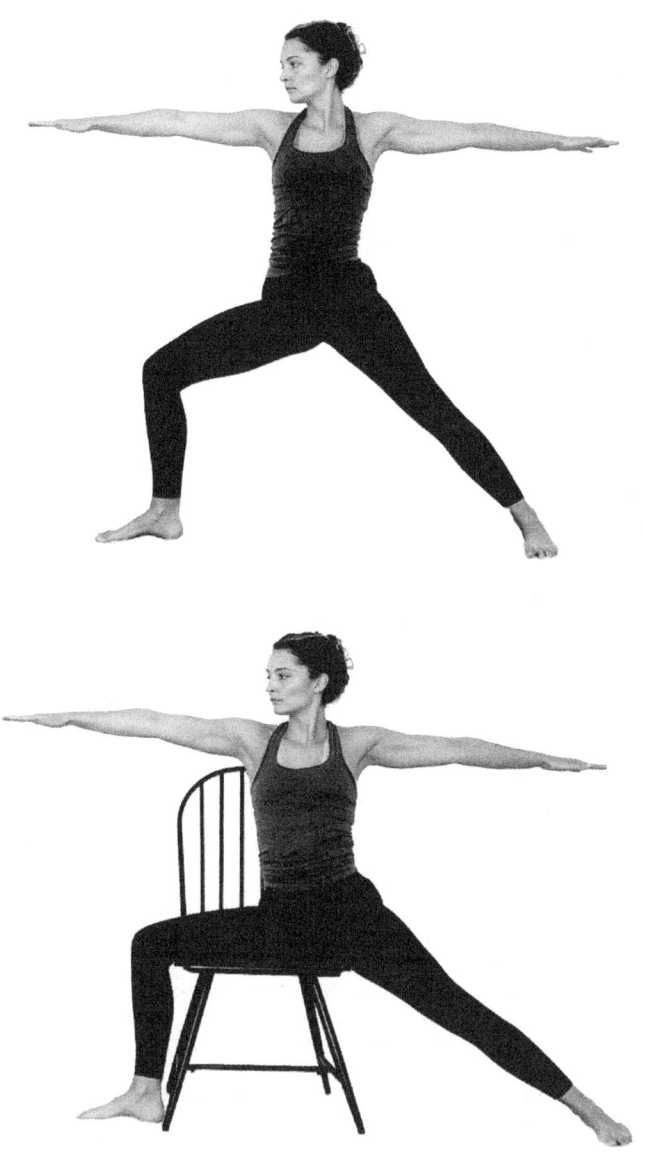

The Plank Poses

Plank Pose on Chair (Phalakasana) #30

While planks are the most doable workouts to strengthen core muscles, a floor plank is still challenging for most of us. I found the chair variation far friendlier and equally effective and realized I could start with this instead of abandoning the pose altogether. Try the upward plank for a more adventurous variation.

SCAN FOR POSE AUDIO

How-to:

1. Stand upright in front of your chair at a distance of about two feet. Bend forward and place your palms on the seat without bending your elbows.
2. Now, walk your legs backward so your legs and spine are in a straight line, like a log leaning forward.
3. Raise your heels so that you are resting on your toes. You will begin to feel a stretch in your calf muscles and hamstring. Keep your core muscles firm and your gaze down, ensuring your neck aligns with your spinal cord.
4.

5. It is important to keep your biceps engaged to prevent your shoulders from sagging.
6. Hold this position for a few breaths while bringing awareness to your entire body.

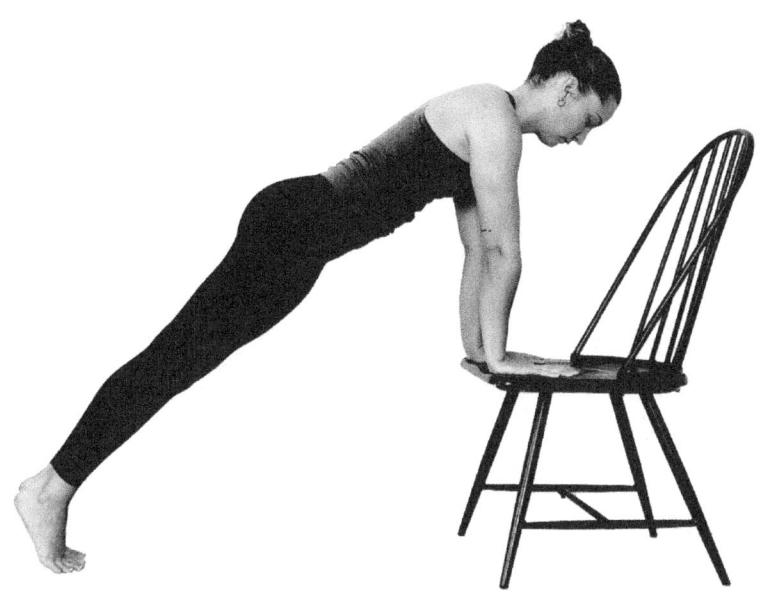

Upward Plank Pose (Upavistha Purvottanasana) #31

This is a good pose for building core muscles, improving arm strength, and ensuring shoulder alignment. It's also beneficial for the thyroid gland and facial muscles.

SCAN FOR POSE AUDIO

How-to:

1. Slide to the front edge of your chair as you extend your legs forward. Your knees should not bend, and your toes should face upward and backward toward you.

2. Focus on your upper body. Take both arms behind you, keep them parallel to each other, and ensure your palms face down with your fingers pointing outward.

3. Look upwards and bend backward slightly. Hold this position for a few seconds. Focus on your breath and feel the sensations of your body.

4. Once you are comfortable with the pose, you can add a variation by lifting your buttocks off the chair and holding the position.

CHAIR YOGA FOR WEIGHT LOSS

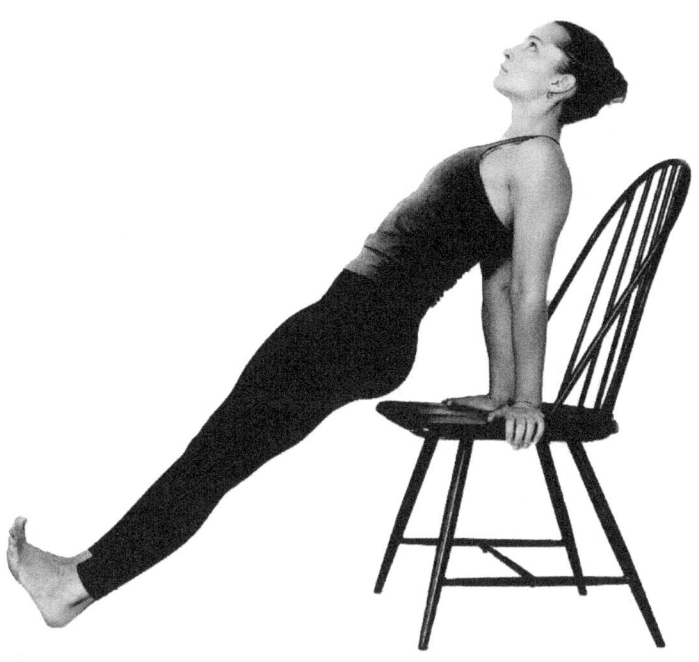

Four-Limbed Staff Pose (Chaturanga Dandasana)

Variation 1 #32

This variation lets you reap the upper body benefits of the *asana*.

SCAN FOR POSE AUDIO

How-to:

1. Sit upright with your feet slightly apart and extend both your arms forward, keeping them parallel to your thighs.
2. Inhale and raise your palms so they face outward. Firm up your arms as if preparing to push an imaginary wall. Hold this position.
3. Exhale while bending your arms at the elbows and bringing them toward you. Hold and repeat.

CHAIR YOGA FOR WEIGHT LOSS

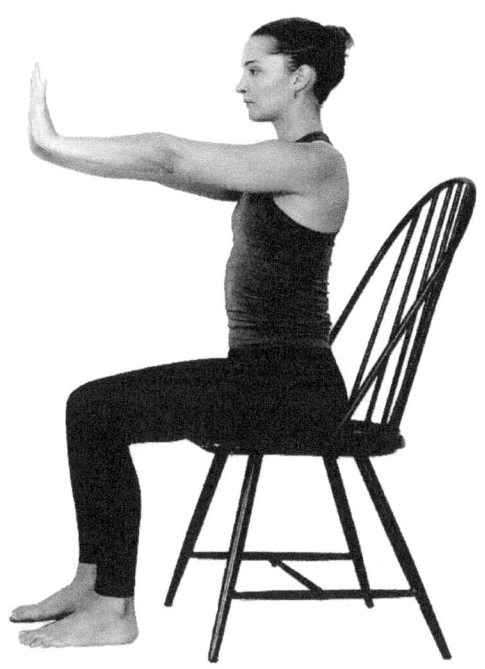

Variation 2 #33

This pose helps achieve an inclined plank by using the chair seat to support your upper body. It works as a safe way of strengthening your arms and wrists.

SCAN FOR POSE AUDIO

How-to:

1. Place your chair against a wall to prevent it from slipping and stand about a foot away, facing the chair.
2. Bend from your knee to place your palms on the chair seat toward the front edge. Walk back to get your arms straight and the weight of your upper body on them. You will begin to feel tension in your upper arms and core. Your knees should have straightened up and your body weight should be on the metatarsals with your heels up in the air.
3. Hold this position and breathe to gain stability. Make sure the crown of your head is in line with your spine.
4. Return to the starting position by walking your legs forward toward the chair. Do a few repetitions.

CHAIR YOGA FOR WEIGHT LOSS

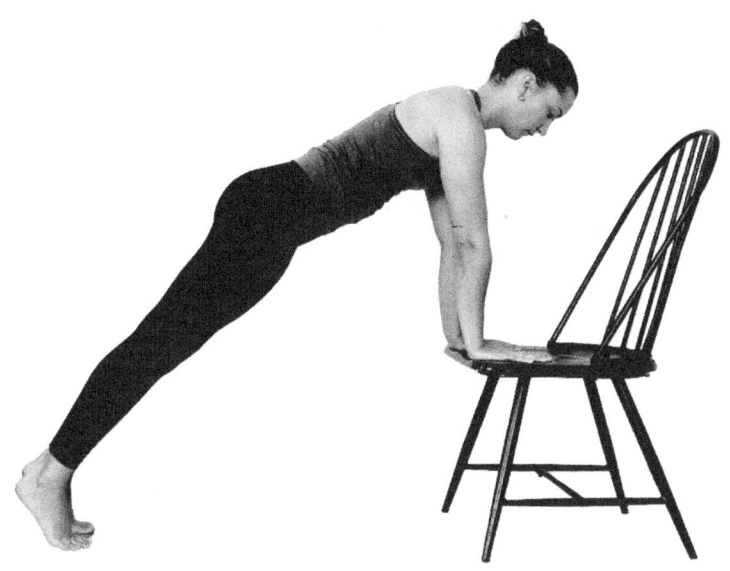

Triangle Pose (Trikonasana) #34

The triangle pose requires you to find a wide stance without bending your knees to form a perfect triangle. The movement of the upper body with the lower body in a triangle position helps improve metabolism by stimulating the digestive organs. It is a fundamental pose that benefits the groin muscles and hamstrings, relieves back stiffness, and is gentle on the body. I found it quite challenging to keep my knees from bending as I began with the upper body movements.

SCAN FOR POSE AUDIO

How-to:

1. Stand upright with a chair on your left side.
2. Spread your legs wide to form a perfect triangle with your toes pointing forward. Place both hands on your waist and hold this position to feel a stretch in your quadriceps and keep your feet well grounded. Your upper body should not wobble.
3. Extend your arms sideways so they are parallel to the ground and at the height of your shoulders.
4. Move your left foot so your toes point outward toward the chair. Keep your right foot at 90 degrees, so your toes are pointed to the sides.

5. Inhale deeply, raise your right hand, placing it against your ear. Exhale and bend your torso to the left.

6. Place your left arm on the chair seat so both arms form a straight line. Keep your gaze towards your right hand.

7. Your knees should not bend at any point. Hold this position for a while before changing sides.

8. It is pertinent to be aware of your spine and sternum positions. They should be expanded to lengthen your upper body.

9. The chair rest helps avoid strain on the waist and encourages you to keep practicing.

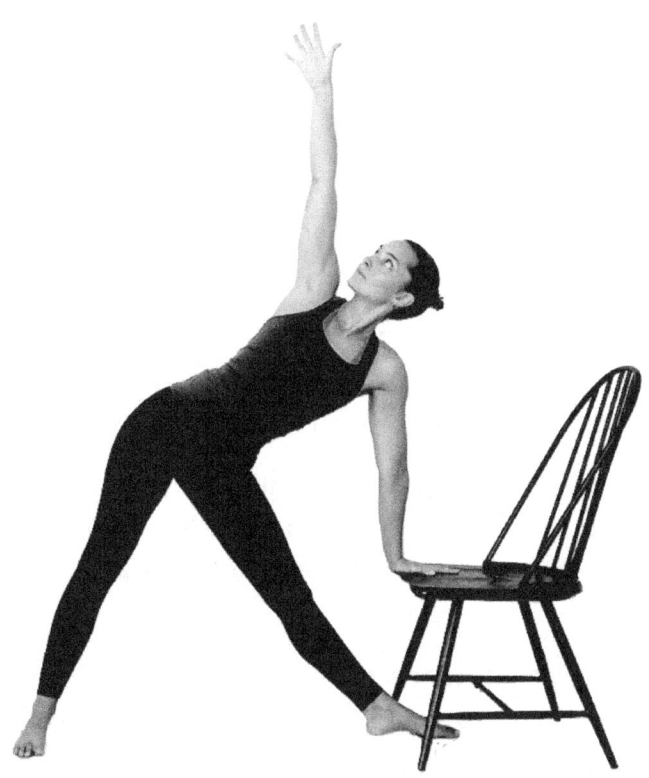

Revolved Triangle Pose (Parivrtta Trikonasana) #35

This pose is based on the triangle pose.

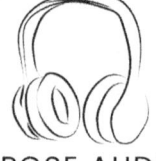

SCAN FOR POSE AUDIO

How-to:

1. Stand upright with a chair on your left side.
2. Spread your legs wide to form a perfect triangle with your toes pointing forward. Place both hands on your waist and hold this position to feel a stretch in your quadriceps and keep your feet well grounded. Your upper body should not wobble.
3. Move your left foot so your toes point outward toward the chair. Move your right foot slightly so your toes point slightly to the left at 45 degrees.
4. As you raise your right hand, rotate your upper body to face your left leg, making sure your hips are squared out.
5. Place your right hand on the seat of the chair. Begin to twist your upper body as you reach your left hand upwards. If it feels okay on your neck, allow your gaze to follow your left hand.
6. You can substitute the chair with a yoga block or stretch to the floor to allow for a deeper bend once you gain more confidence with the stance.

CHAIR YOGA FOR WEIGHT LOSS

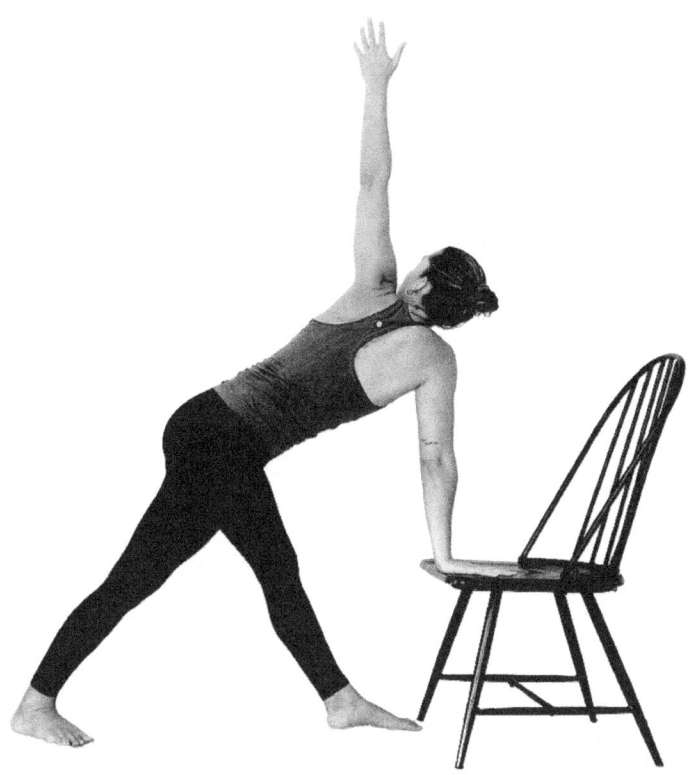

High Lunge Pose and Its Variations

High Lunge Pose With a Chair (Ashta Chandrasana) #36

SCAN FOR POSE AUDIO

How-to:

1. Stand upright in front of your chair. Place your right foot on the chair while taking a deep breath. Your hamstrings should feel a good stretch as you hold the position, and both your legs should be extended away from each other.

2. Exhale while pushing your chest forward and lengthening your spine. See if you can sink a little more into your right leg. Place your hands on your hips as you do so. Hold the high lunge position for four to five long breaths.

3. Release by bringing your right leg down to repeat the pose with your left leg.

CHAIR YOGA FOR WEIGHT LOSS

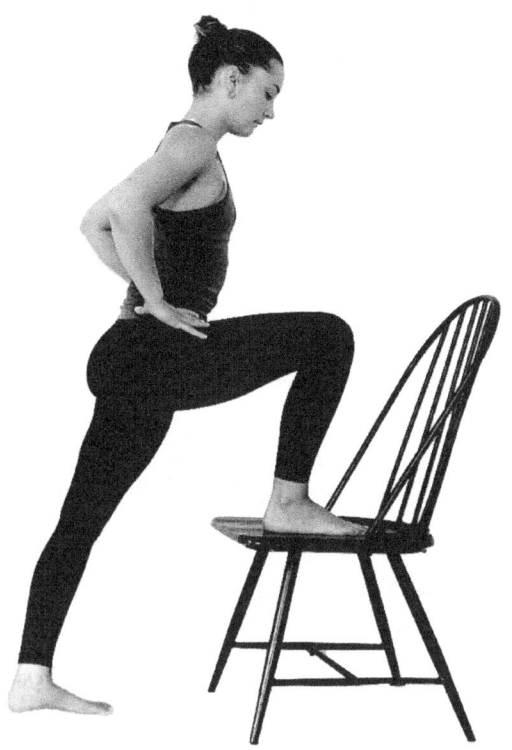

High Lunge Variation (Ashta Chandrasana) #37

SCAN FOR POSE AUDIO

How-to:

1. The same lunge can be achieved by being seated on a chair. Sit upright and spread your legs wide to place your feet well on the sides of your chair.

2. Turn your upper body to the right by shifting your glute muscles, and squaring out your hips. Keep your arms parallel to each other to rest on the seat. Your left leg should be extended straight back with your knee straightening out, grounding through the ball of your foot. Your right leg should be at a 90-degree angle, bent at your knees. Your left leg should be stretched out.

3. Both your hamstrings will benefit from the lunge in this position. Hold the position for a few breaths and repeat on the opposite side.

4. Once you're comfortable with this pose, you can increase difficulty by raising your arms straight above your head and placing your hands in the prayer position.

CHAIR YOGA FOR WEIGHT LOSS

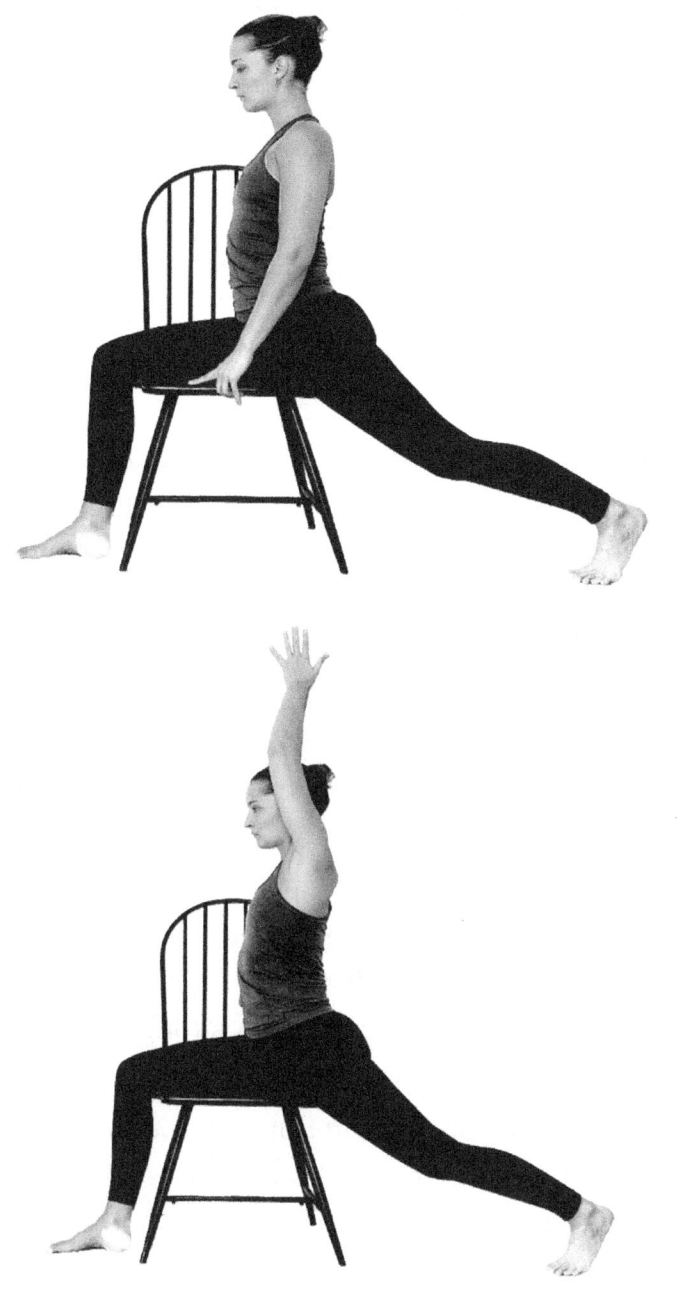

High Lunge Non-Chair (Ashta Chandrasana) #38

SCAN FOR POSE AUDIO

How-to:

1. Stand upright with your legs at least hip-width apart (if not more). Extend your right leg backward with a nice stretch and rest it on your metatarsals with your toes spread wide and heel pointing upward. Check that both feet are in a straight line, one behind the other.

2. Your left leg should maintain a 90-degree bend at your knee with your foot grounded well and toes pointing forward. Your knee should be placed in line with your navel (this is important).

3. Do not let your legs bear the entire weight of your body. Your hip joints and glutes must be equally engaged during the lunge to avoid overstretching your leg muscles. Remember, in this posture, your hips remain strong while your legs indulge in an elaborate stretch.

4. As you stretch your legs, lift both arms to the sides of your ears and keep them parallel with your fingers pointing upward. Keep your chest lifted and open.

5. Your neck should be lengthened, head aligned, and gaze fixed in front. Pull your navel in to engage your core muscles.

6. Hold this position for three to four breaths and repeat on the opposite side. You can increase the count and speed of your repetitions for a more intense workout.

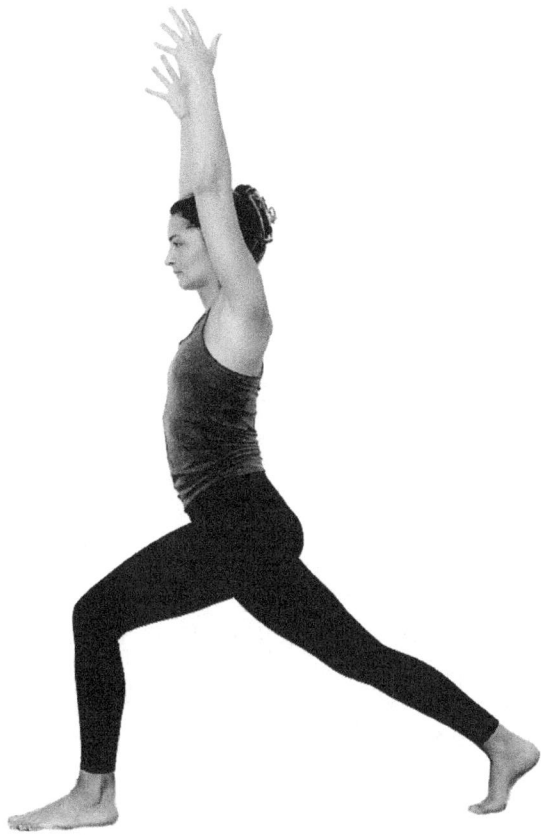

Upward-Facing Dog Pose (Urdhva Mukha Svanasana) #39

SCAN FOR POSE AUDIO

How-to:

1. Stand in front of the chair, seat facing towards you, at a distance that allows you to lean forward and place your hands on the seat.
2. Inhale and bend forward and place the hands on the chair while holding the edges with your palms. Once you get hold of the chair move back with your feet taking the position of the body to about 45 degrees from the ground.
3. Adjusting the legs come to stand on your toes feeling the stretch at the calves, hamstrings and hips..
4. Inhale, and raise your chest up slowly taking the torso in a backbend. Feel the arms and shoulders stretch as the back stretches backwards in a slight backbend.
5. Exhale completely. Inhale to go deeper while making sure the palms are firm on the chair and your toes firm on the ground.
6. Gaze up and back if comfortable and stay for a few breaths while coordinating the breathing process with the stretch.

7. Make sure the shoulders and the wrists are in alignment, make sure the hips move in as you pull the belly in to engage the core muscles. Keep the chest stretched out while taking the shoulders behind.
8. While here, one can keep the feet hip distance apart or depending on the body comfort.
9. Inhale, release the stretch adjusting the hips and legs to get comfortable.

This pose particularly allows you to strengthen your arms while toning the full length of your body.

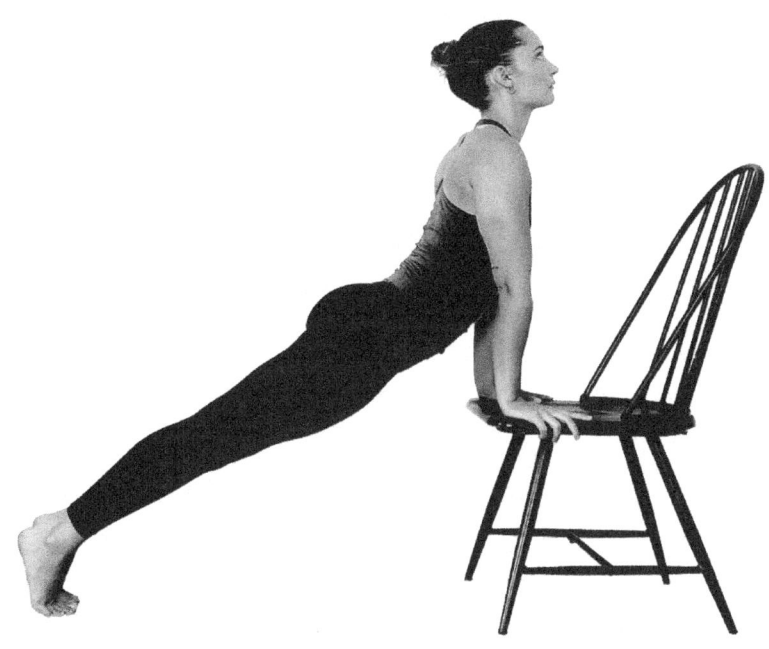

Goddess Pose Side Stretch (Utkata Konasana) #40

This is a side-bend pose that engages your upper body. Spreading your legs in the goddess pose provides a stable base and is a welcome break from the upright positioning of the legs. It provides more stability to maneuver your torso, activates your hips and pelvis area, provides immediate relief from stiff shoulders, and helps ease tension in the mind and body.

SCAN FOR POSE AUDIO

How-to:

1. From the seated mountain pose spread both your legs sideways as much as possible to open your pelvis and hip bones. Keep your feet firmly on the ground and point your toes outward.

2. Focus on your upper body and rest your arms on your thighs with your palms facing up.

3. Take a deep breath while raising your right arm up and sideways over the crown of your head. Your right rib cage will feel a long stretch while the left side of your body remains contracted. Hold this position for five counts and bring your arm and body back to the original position while exhaling well.

4. Repeat on the left side. Alternate and do at least 10 repetitions to benefit from the posture.

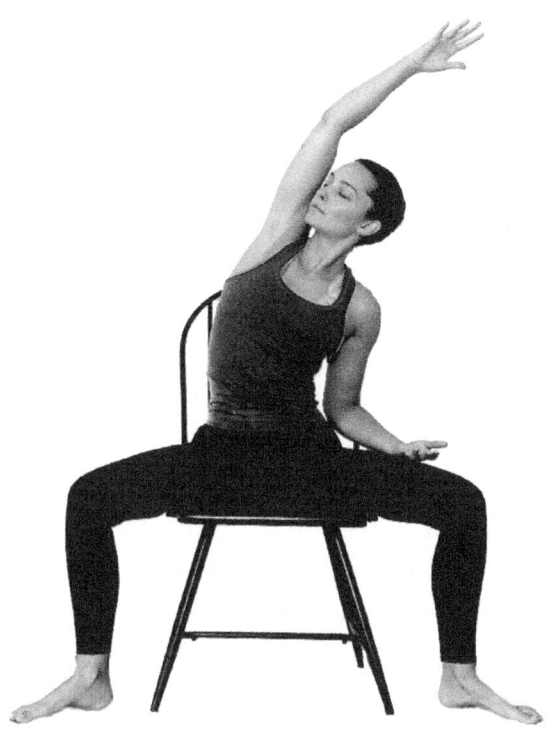

Bharadvaja's Twist (Bharadvajasana) #41

Bharadvaja's Twist is an incredibly satisfying posture in that it massages the spine, neck, and shoulders. Jane specifically asked me to ensure that the twist is felt in the rib area, not in the neck muscles. This pose improves body awareness, helps strengthen your core, and is known to relieve constipation.

SCAN FOR POSE AUDIO

How-to:

1. Sit facing the left side of the chair instead of assuming the usual front-facing stance. Your midriff should be positioned at the center of the backrest so you are neither sitting too much toward the back nor in front of the chair seat.

2. Keep your feet hip-width apart for better balance. Keep both arms by your sides so your palms are in the same direction as your face. Tuck your navel in and keep your spine lengthened.

3. Now, raise both hands to the ceiling, twist your upper body to the right, and place both hands on the backrest, keeping both parallel to each other. You will notice that your left shoulder will stretch more than your right.

4. Hold this position while feeling the pull on the ribs and inhale and exhale for five counts each. Release your grip on the backrest and unwind to repeat on the opposite side.

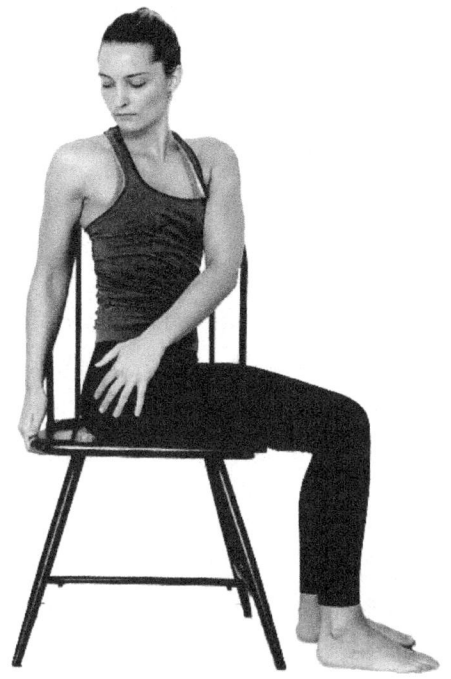

Half-Fish Pose (Ardha Matsyendrasana) #42

SCAN FOR POSE AUDIO

How-to:

1. Assume the *Easy Pose* stance on the chair (or on the floor) with both legs folded in an easy pose. Now, cross your right leg over your left and place your right foot snugly next to your left hip while ensuring your right knee faces the ceiling. Take time to feel the stretch of your glutes.

2. Place your right hand on the seat for support and check for balance. You should be distributing your weight on both hip bones.

3. Raise your left hand toward the ceiling and bring it down to place your elbow on the outside of your right knee. Keep them pressed together so they don't slip off from their position. This will force your triceps and left rib cage to stretch.

4. Turn your gaze to the right, gently looking past your right shoulder without straining your neck and lock your gaze at a comfortable distance.

5. Inhale and exhale with each new position to feel its sensations.
6. Hold this position for five counts and gradually release your gaze, hands, and legs to return to the *Easy Pose*.

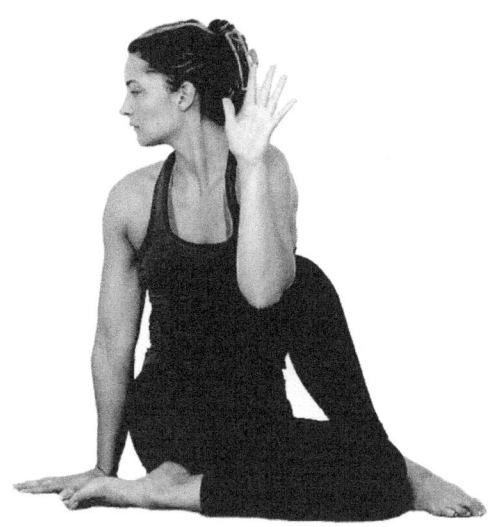

Vishnu's Couch Pose (Ananthasana) #43

This pose tremendously improves balance and strengthens the nervous system. Apart from providing a good stretch to the torso and hamstrings, it helps reduce obesity in the thigh and hip region when done regularly. The pose is used as a form of therapy to reduce lower back pain but cannot be done if one has cervical spondylitis or a slipped disc.

SCAN FOR POSE AUDIO

How-to:

1. Lie down on your left side on a yoga mat or carpet. Support your head with your left hand by resting your triceps on the ground and bending your arm at the elbow to allow your head to rest on your palm. Your right leg will rest on the left.

2. Place your right hand in front of your chest to feel well-balanced. Hold this position and take a few deep breaths to feel the sensations from head to toe.

3. Slowly raise your right leg without bending your knee and try to keep it vertical to the ground. You will feel a stretch in your pelvis and glutes. Inhale while raising and exhale while you bring your leg back to the resting position.

4. Once you get better at raising your leg (and this may take quite a few days of practice), take your right hand off the

ground since you will now use your hand to support your raised leg.

5. Bend your right leg toward your pelvis and hold your big toe with your right-hand thumb, pointer, and middle finger.

6. Gently raise your leg to a vertical position, stretching it up with your right hand until your hand and leg are at a perfect right angle to the ground. Hold this position for a few breaths and then return to the resting position by releasing your leg.

7. To change directions, sit up by raising your upper body first, take the Easy Pose, and repeat on the opposite side.

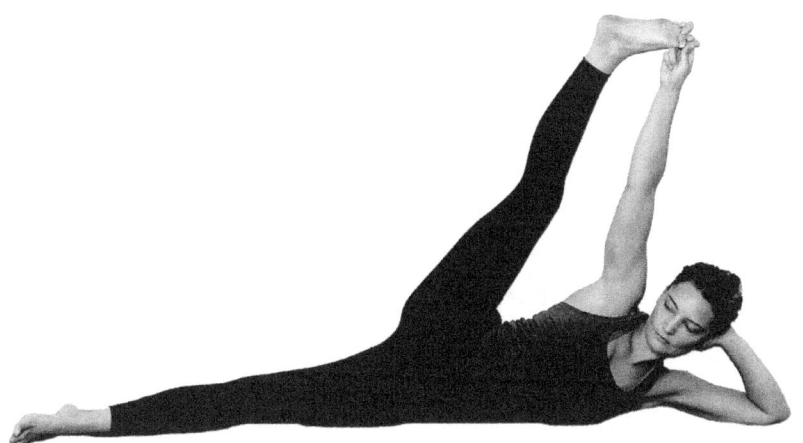

Half Frog Pose (Ardha Bhekasana) #44

SCAN FOR POSE AUDIO

How-to:

1. Lie down on the ground on your belly. It's best to start with the downward dog pose and proceed to lie flat on the ground.

2. Lift your upper body by pressing your forearms to the ground with your elbows bent and underneath your shoulders. Your arms should be shoulder-width apart with your fingers pointing forward.

3. Your sternum should be almost vertical, and your collarbones should be broadened to open your chest. Try to keep your naval up, not resting on the floor.

4. Your toes should rest on the floor while your heels point to the ceiling. Face forward at all times.

5. Once you feel stable on your belly with your chest opened up, lift your right leg by bending your knee so that your foot reaches your glutes.

6. Move your right arm simultaneously to be able to hold your right foot. Your palm should grasp the upper side of your foot. You will feel a pull on your biceps and triceps as you do so.

7. Keep your foot slightly pressed and check your position for balance. Your shoulders, back, and chest should not feel unduly strained.

You will feel your quadriceps stretching as you deepen the press of your foot with your hand. If your quads are flexible, you can deepen the bend until your toes rest next to your waist and your elbows point to the ceiling. Ensure your chest remains lifted as you hold the position for around six to eight breaths. Release your right leg and repeat with your left leg.

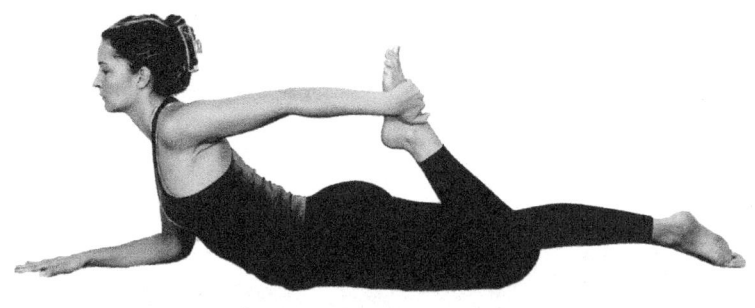

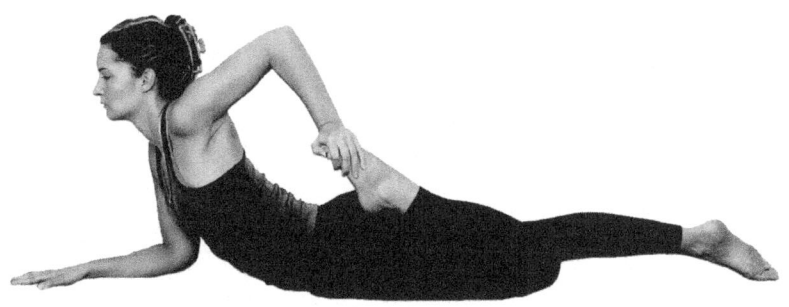

Half Frog Variation With a Strap #45

If you find it difficult to bend your legs in the prone position, loop a yoga strap or rolled-up towel around your feet to pull them toward your glutes.

 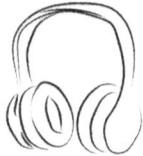

SCAN FOR POSE AUDIO

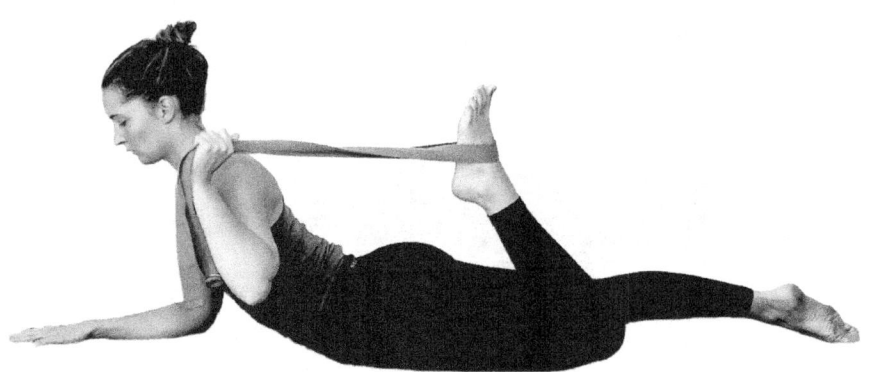

Pyramid Pose (Parsvottanasana) #46

SCAN FOR POSE AUDIO

How-to:

1. On the yoga mat, stand upright with your legs spread hip-width apart, hands placed beside your hips, and palms facing forward. Keep your shoulders rolled back and spine straight. Inhale and exhale a few times to feel your body from head to toe.

2. Next, place your right foot back comfortably and line up the heels of both your feet on an imaginary line passing vertically through where you are standing. Make sure your back foot is rotated at 45 degrees, with your toes pointed out slightly. Your feet should be about three feet apart at all times.

3. Press down the soles of both your feet to the ground for stability. You may feel a little wobble while your body achieves balance. Place your hands on your hips for better control and keep your thighs engaged at all times.

4. Inhale deeply and spread your arms to the side. Exhale while turning your palms and bending your elbows to bring your forearms behind you in the reverse prayer position. If you find it difficult to put your palms together behind your

back, grab opposite forearms behind your back, or keep your arms down alongside your hips.

5. Setting a chair in front of you will help because you can place your hands in front of the seat during the forward fold.

6. Another option is to set two blocks in front of you and place your hands on them as you fold forward.

7. Bend forward so your upper body is parallel to the ground. Keep your arms connected behind your back, or if that is initially difficult rest your hands on the back of the chair, the chair seat, or the yoga blocks, depending on your flexibility. With practice, you will be able to bend forward from your hips so your upper body folds forward deeply and your face touches your knees.

8. Resisting the urge to bend your knee is a task in itself. Keeping your thigh muscles taut and hips engaged will help. Focus on the hamstring of your forward leg. It gets the most stretching, and this knowledge will keep you from bending your knee.

9. You will need to keep both feet firmly on the ground at all times to help maintain stability.

10. Hold this position and release by inhaling and bringing your upper body gently back to an upright position.

CHAIR YOGA FOR WEIGHT LOSS

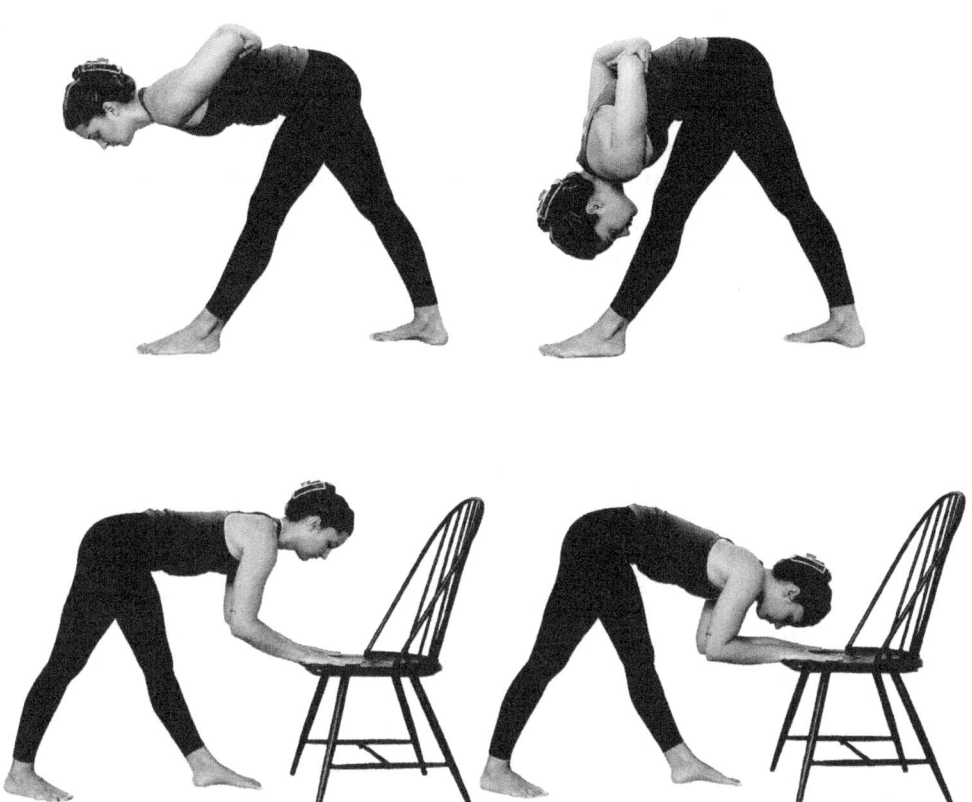

Dancer's Pose (Natarajasana) #47

When Jane finally was confident that I would stick with yoga, she revealed more postures like a magician pulling seemingly never-ending tricks out of their hat. The dancer's pose was one such trick that got me excited on Sunday morning. The morning dew on my bare feet and the much-awaited sighting of the red-tailed hawks busy nesting at the park already made me want to dance with abandon.

The dancer's pose is a deep backbend and demands a steady sense of calm. You start by warming up your shoulders, hips, and thighs for a smooth experience. Since it requires balancing on one leg, you need to be more alert and not overly tired. Placing a chair in front of you will provide the necessary support until you feel comfortable enough to attempt it without a chair around. Your ankles benefit, you feel more balanced, and your hip flexors, quadriceps, and glute muscles are engaged.

SCAN FOR POSE AUDIO

How-to:

1. Stand upright behind a chair with the backrest facing you. Keep your rib cage and sternum relaxed. With a slight thrust, lift your right leg behind you.

2. Bend your right knee and place your heel behind your right glute. Simultaneously, reach your right arm back and clasp your right ankle firmly.
3. Press your left leg to the ground firmly and gently hold the chair's backrest with your left arm.
4. Hold this position for six to eight counts to observe your body and check your overall posture. You should feel stable at this point. Your upper body will slightly thrust forward.
5. When you feel more confident, avoid holding on to the chair and raise your left arm to match the angle of your right arm. You will feel like a dancer in control!
6. Release your leg to repeat on the opposite side.

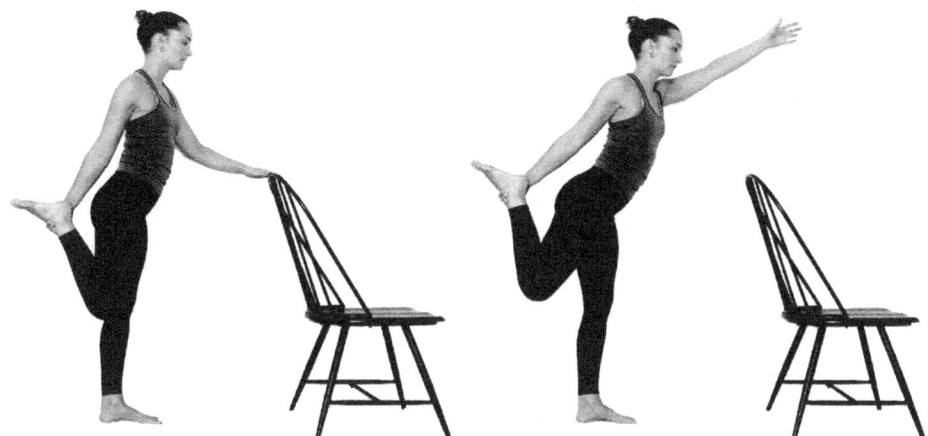

The Garland Pose (Malasana) and Its Variations

The garland pose has wonderful variations of wide-footed deep squats. Squatting has unfortunately become a lost art since the invention of the chair. It came naturally to us as children and was abandoned once we were presented with a chair.

Farmers and people who perform physical labor get into this position more often. Start squatting if you want to protect your future mobility and experience the benefits it can bring you.

Years of not squatting led to a limited range of motion in my lower body. This pose is not advisable if you have a significant knee or back injury; otherwise, it can be gradually internalized without any problem. Some people find it easier, as body proportions have a role to play. Jane mentioned how people with a longer torso generally have it easier.

The garland pose is to be initially mastered with the help of props like a towel, bolster, chair, or hubby (yes, they are sometimes effective) and then performed on the floor without aid. This progression will be one hell of a show of self-love. This pose opens up your hips and groin and vitalizes your feet and ankles. Let us look at its progressions and variations one by one.

Seated Garland Pose (Upavistha Malasana) #48

SCAN FOR POSE AUDIO

How-to:

1. Use a bolster or yoga blocks beneath your feet to get the required elevation. Sit upright, deep into the chair, with your hands resting on your thighs while you focus on your breath.

2. Rest your feet firmly on the bolster or yoga blocks and touch the chair's front legs. Keep your feet moderately apart near the edges of the bolster. Adjust your hips, thighs, and lower back. Tuck your navel in to keep your belly engaged at all times.

3. Bring your palms to the prayer position in front of your chest and lean forward so that your elbows touch the chair's seat from in between your spread-out thighs.

4. Ensure your chest is kept broad and your shoulders rolled back to prevent your upper body from drooping. Your gaze can be kept locked in front.

5. Hold this position and move your torso forward for a deeper stretch with each exhalation. Relax with every inhalation and bend forward with each exhalation for perfect coordination. You will feel an evident relaxation in your hips and groin muscles.

6. Come out of the pose by getting your feet off the bolster and back to an upright position with your feet hip-width apart.

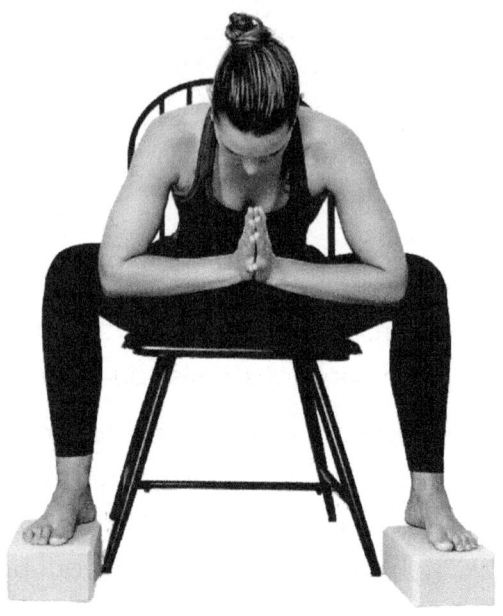

Garland Pose Hands-On Chair Support (Malasana Hasta) #49

Once you get a feel of how *malasana* works on a chair, you can try it on the floor using the chair for upper body support.

SCAN FOR POSE AUDIO

How-to:

1. Place a chair facing you about two feet in front.

2. Stand upright and spread your feet so they are more than hip-width apart, toes point outward slightly. Bend forward and hold the chair seat to resemble the downward dog pose.

3. Your shoulders should not droop. Your navel should be tucked in. Your core muscles should be firm. Breathe to feel the sensations in your pelvis.

4. Gently lower yourself to the ground and push your hips down as much as you can. Your toes will tend to point away from each other. Ensure your spine is lengthened and your shoulders are pulled away from your ears.

5. You will notice your upper body pushing forward a bit. Take care not to let it push forward so much that your knees move below hip level, which would be an incorrect posture.

6. Hold this position. It will initially feel very taxing for your lower body but get better with practice.

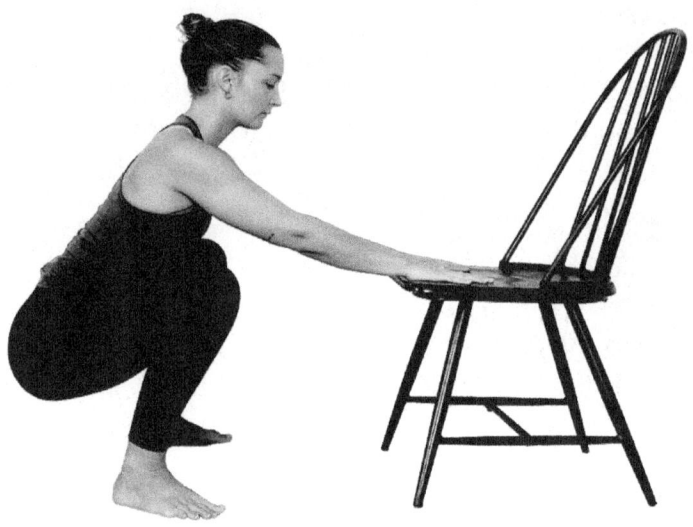

Garland Pose With Towel, Blocks, or a Partner #50

The concept of *malasana* can feel weird for someone unfamiliar with the pose. It requires a certain flexibility of the ankles, knees, pelvis, hips, and spine that can take time to develop.

Your ankle joints can have a hard time if you are not used to the pose. However, this shouldn't prevent you from trying to do it.

SCAN FOR POSE AUDIO

How-to:

1. Lay a rolled-up towel on the floor and place your heels on it to relieve your joints when your entire body weight falls on them. This greatly helps you avoid falls and balance your body when squatting.
2. Alternatively, place a yoga block behind you so that your glute muscles rest on it when you squat. This will support your quadriceps and pelvis, thus encouraging you to continue practicing.
3. For a fun variation, have a partner hold your hands and get into the garland position together. Practicing with your partner will help strengthen the pose and your relationship as a bonus.

4. Regular practice will build strength in your ankles and flexibility in your lower body, giving you the confidence to do away with props.

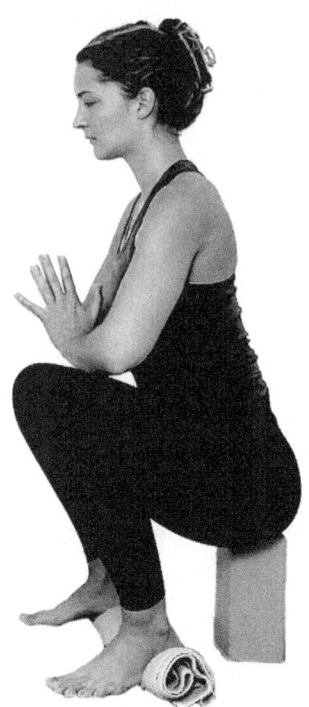

Garland Pose (Malasana) #51

When you feel ready to do a classic *malasana*, try the following positions:

SCAN FOR POSE AUDIO

How-to:

1. Start by squatting and keep your hands in a prayer position with your elbows touching your knees from the inside and pushing them apart.
2. Your shoulder blades should be away from each other and your spine should be lengthened to a slight forward bend.
3. Your hips and sitting bones should be lifted and thrust toward the ground.
4. Your chest should not droop. Keep your chin lifted and away from your chest so your gaze is in front of you.
5. Your core should be engaged with your navel tucked in.
6. Your knees should point up and away from each other and your feet should be grounded firmly with your ankle joints bearing weight. Keep your toes pointed a bit outward for good balance.

THE MAYA METHOD

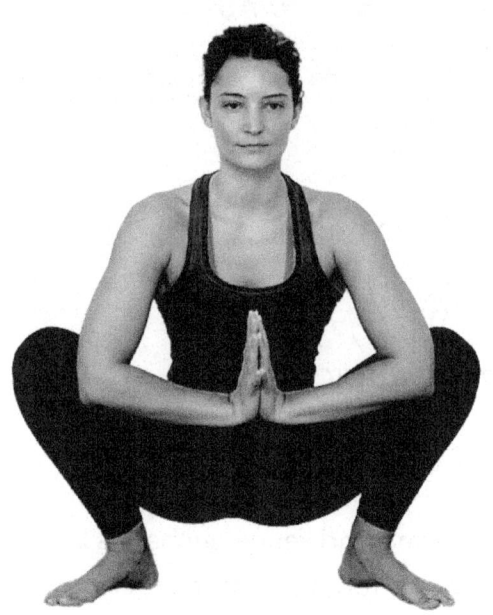

Garland Half Broken Wing Pose (Malasana Ardha Avabhinna Pakshasana) #52

This pose is a progression that lets you celebrate your ability to perform a deep squat on the floor.

SCAN FOR POSE AUDIO

How-to:

1. Get into the squatting position with your thighs wide open. Spread your bent knees and legs wide. Keep your buttocks lifted off the floor at all times.

2. Place your arms on the side of your waist for stability.

3. Gently move your right hand onto your right knee and your upper body away toward the left while straightening your right arm. Your heel may lift during this movement—that's fine. Take time to adjust and find complete harmony in this pose.

4. Keep your gaze on your right hand placed on your knee. Hold the position for about 10 breaths.

5. To release, place your right arm back on your waist and repeat on the opposite side so that you devote an equal number of stretches to both sides.

6. To release the garland pose, place your palms on the floor and raise your hips to straighten your legs to an upright position without any sudden movements.

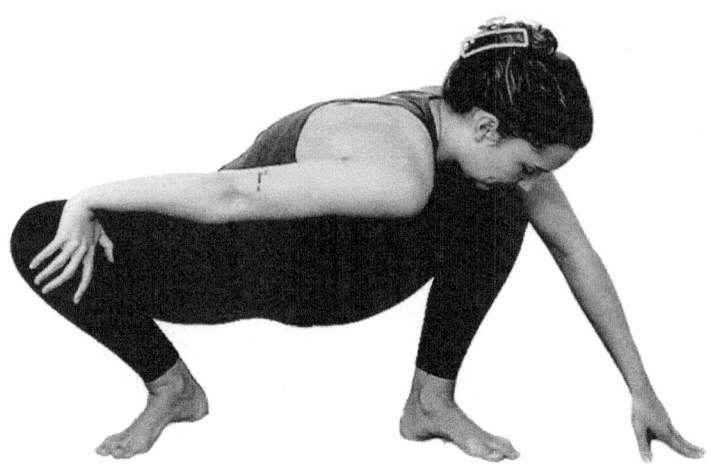

Revolved Chair Pose (Parivrtta Utkatasana) #53

The revolved chair pose must be attempted only after a few solid months of flexing your body with the basic postures. I remember feeling lightheaded while my shoulder blades beseeched for help the first time I tried it. But with patience, you will learn to make friends with the pose and harness the energy it generously gives you.

This pose can be done by sitting on a real or imaginary chair from the standing position. The fact that you need to balance and twist makes this a special experience. Over time, this pose has helped my ankles move better and my upper body feel unblocked with all the twists.

SCAN FOR POSE AUDIO

How-to:

1. Stand upright with a chair ready behind you. Keep your feet slightly apart for better balance.
2. Inhale deeply and raise your arms along your ears and over your head.
3. Exhale, bend your knees, and thrust your hips down to sit on the chair. If you decide not to use a chair, you need to imagine a chair and let your glute muscles sit in thin air.

4. Notice how your body weight will shift to your heel when there is no chair. Do not let your chest and abdomen cave in at this stage.

5. Keep your knees apart at the same distance as your ankles and tighten your quadriceps.

6. Inhale deeply while bringing your hands in front of your chest in a prayer position. Keep your elbow away from your rib cage and stretch upward to lengthen your spinal cord.

7. Exhale and bend your upper body downward toward the right to rest your left elbow on the outside of your right knee. This deep twist will challenge your shoulder blades and neck. If you're doing it without a chair, don't let your knees move in front of your toes at any point, as this will cause your weight to shift toward the front.

8. Be steady in your movements and bring your gaze behind you in line with your right elbow. Your elbow has to be visible to you and should not be pushed behind your back. Check if your knees are in line with each other since there's a tendency for one knee to move forward, which needs to be avoided.

9. Hold this position for about six breaths if possible and release, returning to an upright position to repeat on the opposite side.

CHAIR YOGA FOR WEIGHT LOSS

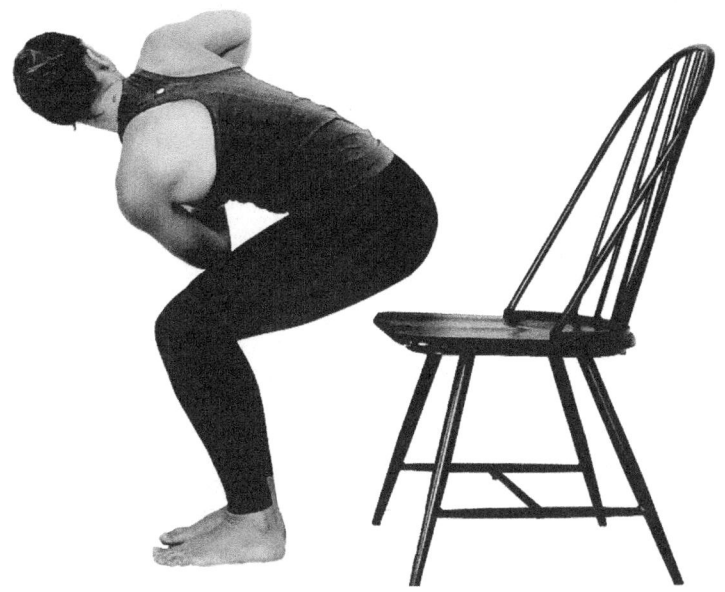

Revolved Chair Pose Variation (Parivrtta Utkatasana Variation) #54

SCAN FOR POSE AUDIO

How-to:

1. Stand upright with a chair ready behind you. Keep your feet slightly apart for better balance.
2. Inhale deeply and raise your arms along your ears and over your head.
3. Exhale, bend your knees, and thrust your hips down to sit on the chair. If you decide not to use a chair, you need to imagine a chair and let your glute muscles sit in thin air.
4. From the seated position bend down and place your right hand on the outside of your left foot.
5. Raise your left arm towards the ceiling so that both your arms are in a straight line. Try to follow your gaze to the tip of your left arm. This could be challenging, as it could initially strain your left shoulder.
6. Hold this position for five counts and gently lower your extended arm before returning to an upright position. Repeat on the opposite side.

CHAIR YOGA FOR WEIGHT LOSS

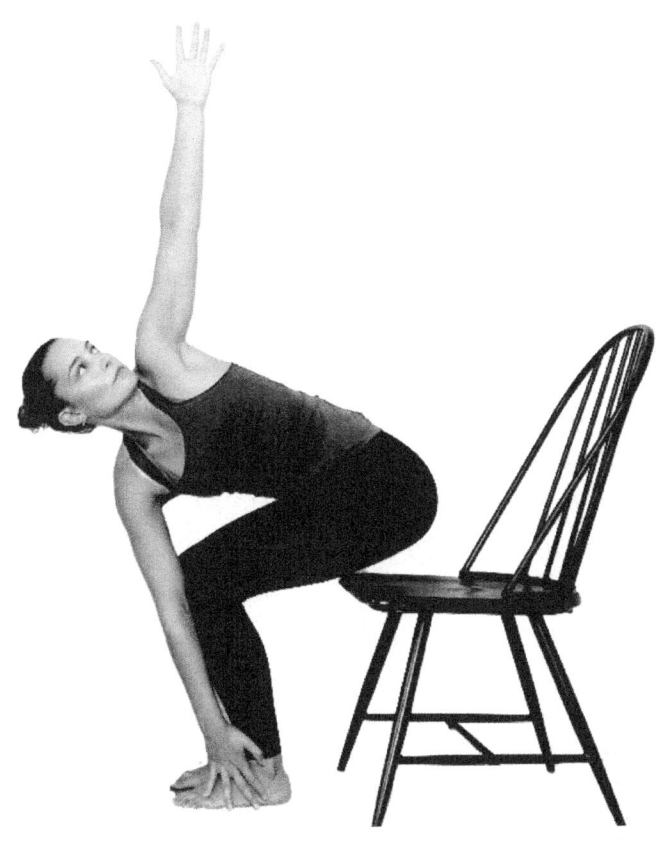

Half Moon Pose on Chair (Ardha Chandrasana) #55

Wobble, wobble, wobble... is how I went during the initial days of practice, and that's how it goes even today if I don't precede it with warm-up and foundational poses. Spend time on the hip-relaxing and hamstring-stretching beginner poses before getting into this one; this holds true even for experts. Don't get carried away with the seemingly straightforward how-to instructions for this!

The half-moon and the sugarcane bow pose are intermediate-level postures that call for a confident side bend. I ventured to do it only after I gained some confidence in understanding my body's capacity to flex and balance itself. Pushing too fast can invite cramps in your thigh muscles. Only when I got deeper into its practice did I begin to perceive the sense of stability it brought.

SCAN FOR POSE AUDIO

How-to:

1. Stand in front of your chair facing the seat rest at an arm's length distance. Raise your arms, tuck your navel in, and bend forward to rest your forearms on the seat. Check for stability by placing your feet at hip-width distance.

2. Now, extend your right leg back to rest on your toes while slightly bending your left knee. As you check the alignment

of your shoulders, forearms, hips, and knees, hold your position for a few breaths.

3. Gently lift your right leg off the floor, keeping it parallel to the floor while straightening your left knee. You won't be able to keep your leg parallel without weeks of practice. Your groin muscles will need some serious training.

4. Adjust the position of your left foot so that your ankle can bear your full body weight. Focus on every sensation.

5. Once you gain confidence with leg positions, raise your right hand from your chair rest. Place it on your hips first to check for stability. Then gently raise it upward while turning your torso to the right. The right side of your hips will also be lifted in the process.

6. Shift your gaze up to look at the fingers on your right arm. This step will need patient practice before it comes naturally.

7. You should be able to achieve this by shifting your body weight on your left arm and shoulders in the process, which is the challenge.

8. Keep your left foot grounded well, chest expanded, and core muscles taut. Maintain the pose for about six breaths and repeat on the opposite side.

THE MAYA METHOD

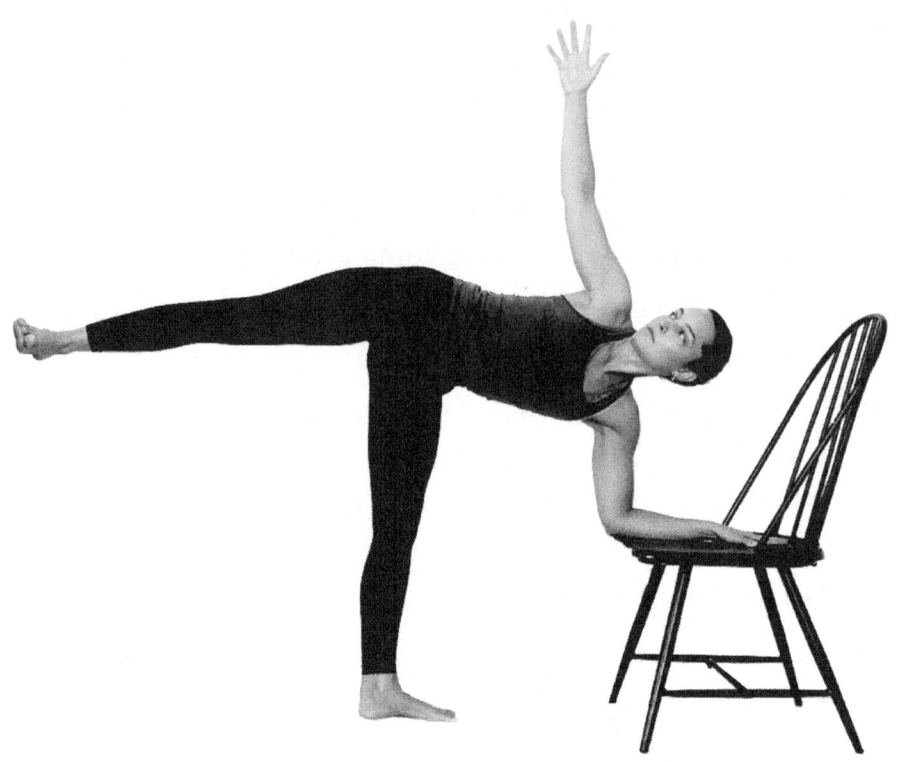

Sugarcane Bow Pose on Chair (Ardha Chandra Chapasana) #56

This pose is for those brave souls who want to go beyond the half moon pose.

SCAN FOR POSE AUDIO

How-to:

1. Get into the half moon pose even if it takes a month. If your right leg is stretched out, fold it into your chest by bringing in your right knee. Your right hand should clutch the top of your right foot.

2. Once you feel stable in this position, lead your right foot behind you by swinging your knee behind you. Push your foot forward into your hands to spread out fully.

3. Stay in this hard-earned position and ensure your shoulders, upper body, and right thigh are in a straight line. If they are not, you'll invite unwarranted strains, and we are not looking for trouble. Hold for a few breaths to feel the strength of your body.

4. Release your leg first and return to the upright position to repeat on the opposite side.

THE MAYA METHOD

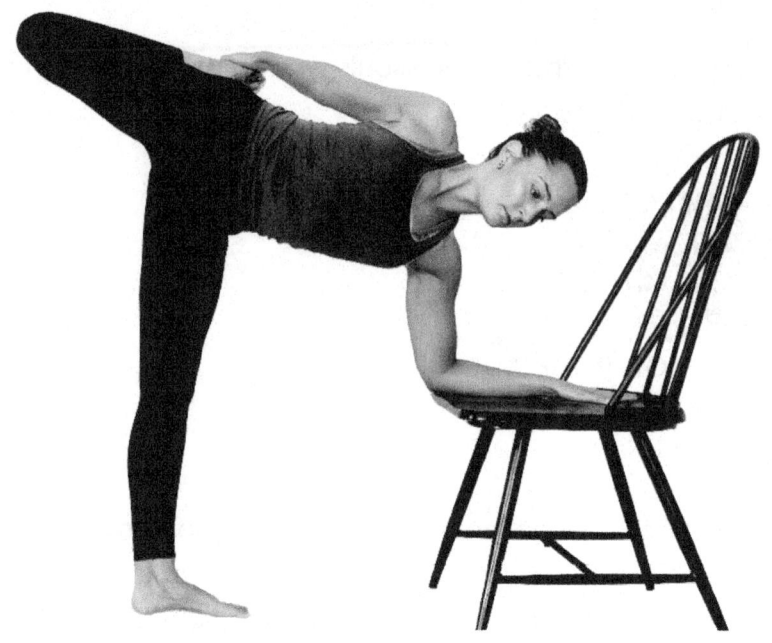

Bound Angle and Seated Upward Straddle Pose (Baddha Konasana and Urdhva Upavistha Konasana) #57

I spent months getting used to sitting cross-legged on my chair and the floor before I could try the bound angle pose. The upward straddle looks like an out-of-bound aspiration but is worth trying nevertheless. I would save it for the end of my yoga sequences even after months of practice. Since the poses require fairly loosened hamstrings and groin muscles, it's best to do enough of the foundational poses laid out in the beginning.

SCAN FOR POSE AUDIO

How-to:

1. Sit upright toward the front of the seat. Spread out your feet nice and wide to straddle. Keep your hands behind your glute muscles and parallel to each other with your fingers pointing backward.

2. Lift up your right leg by bending your knee and bringing your foot to the middle of the chair just below your navel. Feel the muscle stretch in the middle of your back and be mindful of all muscle stretches to avoid undue strains.

3. Bring your left foot up similarly so that both your soles touch each other. Roll your shoulders back and lengthen your spine so your sitting bones settle and your thighs remain grounded on the chair seat. This is the bound angle pose. Stay in the position for a few breaths and relax.

4. Take time to get used to this since your groin muscles must be activated. Everyday practice will help you get comfortable.

5. Achieving the straddle will initially look tricky and require patience and focus. At the bound angle pose, bring your arms to the front and hold your big toes by locking your thumb with your pointer and middle fingers.

6. Roll your shoulders back and gently lift your feet off the seat with a slight backward bend of your upper body so that it touches the backrest.

7. Now, extend your legs outward and upward using your hands to provide the lift.

8. Getting your legs to stretch out straight away will undoubtedly be a tall order. Even if they are bent at your knees and have not moved wide enough, it is not fair to despair.

9. Keep your spine and tailbone lengthened and your sitting bones grounded well. Hold this pose for as long as you can and return to the crossed legs position to relax. Your hamstrings will take time to break in—that's perfectly alright.

CHAIR YOGA FOR WEIGHT LOSS

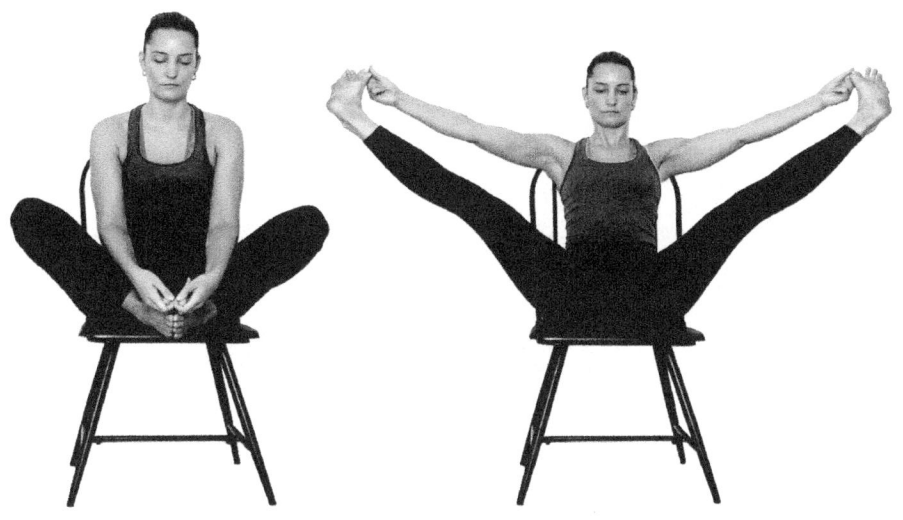

If you wish to broaden your training to include resistance band exercises and High Intensity Interval Training (HIIT) download your **Free Bonus**.

SCAN TO DOWNLOAD BONUS

CONCLUSION

We hope that Maya's accounts of her discoveries light a spark in each one of us. Her life situations are unique to her, and her inferences are but the results of a combination of factors that define her environment. Your journey is unique. It's just that it helps when we remind each other that we have a common thread that binds us together despite all the diversity. Our intents, emotions, and fundamental principles of well-being tie us together in trials and victories.

Thus, when the done list in your weekly workout calendar reflects a combination of exercises to account for aerobic drills, strength training, and flexibility, you will know you are on the right path. When you find a pleasurable workout session that uses good technique and discipline, you will know it's a keeper. When your days have a healthy combination of rest and hard work, you will know your routine is sustainable. When your plate contains high-quality nourishment and invites you to eat with mindfulness, you will know you have found your secret to being in top form.

We loved Maya's discoveries, and we can't wait to hear yours!

Dear Reader,

To download your Free Bonus Material:

- **Resistance Band Exercises** and **HIIT Workout Book**
- Maya's favorite **Five Yoga Sequences** (flows) plus
- Register to receive a **free digital copy of Maya's next book** scan the QR code below:

SCAN FOR A FREE BONUS

We have a favor to ask:

If you enjoyed Maya story please take a couple of minutes to write a short review on Amazon? We'll be checking the reviews personally and your honest feedback will help others understand how they will benefit from Maya's Method.

Reviews are the life blood for indie authors attempting to compete with established publishing houses and their large advertising budgets.

SCAN TO LEAVE A REVIEW

Thank you!

Florence and David

Made in United States
Orlando, FL
24 January 2025